DISCOVER THE NATURAL MEDICINE
ALTERNATIVE FOR . . .

ANXIETY DISORDERS

Complete relaxation and its healing attributes can be gained from **tai chi chuan,** and practicing this artful exercise for twenty minutes each day not only has a calming effect on your mind and nervous system, it can rejuvenate your body and prolong your life.

MOOD DISORDERS

Conventional medicine can break the cycle of persistent, recurrent, and severe episodes of depression, but **acupuncture** balances the flow of *chi* and blood throughout your body and can help resolve the underlying energy imbalance contributing to your depression.

DAILY STRESS

To induce calm and treat everyday stress or mental fatigue, **aromatherapy** can provide near instant relief, and it's simple! Just dip cotton in such essences as a mixture of lavender, geranium, and patchouli for tension and anxiety; chamomile and melissa for an antispasmodic and nerve sedative.

PLUS . . .

**TENSION HEADACHES • EYESTRAIN • PANIC ATTACKS
PHOBIAS • OBSESSIVE-COMPULSIVE DISORDER
POSTTRAUMATIC STRESS DISORDER • SLEEPLESSNESS
SEASONAL AFFECTIVE DISORDER (SAD)**

THE DELL NATURAL MEDICINE LIBRARY
Health and Healing the Natural Way

LOOK FOR THESE OTHER TITLES IN
THE DELL NATURAL MEDICINE LIBRARY:

Women's Health
Chronic Pain
Asthma and Allergies

THE NATURAL WAY
OF HEALING

STRESS, ANXIETY, AND DEPRESSION

The Natural Medicine Collective

Dr. Brian Fradet, D.C.
(Coordinating Panelist, Chiropractic)
Dr. William Bergman, M.D. *(Homeopathy)*
Brian Clement *(Nutrition)*
Elaine Retholtz, L.Ac. *(Acupuncture)*
Dr. James Lawrence Thomas, Ph.D. *(Psychology)*
Dr. Maurice H. Werness, Jr., N.D. *(Naturopathy)*

with
Diana L. Ajjan

A DELL BOOK

PRODUCED BY THE PHILIP LIEF GROUP, INC.

Published by
Dell Publishing
a division of
Bantam Doubleday Dell Publishing Group, Inc.
1540 Broadway
New York, New York 10036

Note to the Reader:

This book is not for the purpose of self-diagnosis or self-treatment, and should be used only in conjunction with the advice of your personal doctor. Readers should consult an appropriate medical professional in all matters relating to their health.

Produced by The Philip Lief Group, Inc., 6 West 20th Street, New York, New York

ISBN: 978-0-440-61403-6

Published simultaneously in Canada

144915995

Contents

THE NATURAL WAY
OF HEALING

STRESS, ANXIETY, AND DEPRESSION

Introduction

Life is a state of mind . . . age is a state of mind
. . . health is a state of mind . . . According to these
well-worn phrases, the mind bears an enormous responsibility in this world. Indeed, it is the essence of life and it
determines an individual's well-being, or health.

Natural medicine offers a variety of therapies for different kinds of illness. What they all share, and what sets
them apart from conventional medicine, is a holistic approach. Physicians of natural medicine consider the whole
person—mind and body—in the diagnosis and treatment
of patients, and their therapies also respect this integra-
tion.

Considering the emphasis on the mind/body connection, natural medicine therapies can be effective in treating illnesses of the mind, such as anxiety disorders and
depression. The most important goal is to care for the
mind *before* illness develops. A strong positive mental attitude promotes a healthier body. Together, a healthy mind
and body allow an individual to experience life to the full-
est and to achieve self-actualization. This concept, advocated by the humanist psychologist Abraham Maslow, refers to a person's potential to accomplish his or her
dreams, wishes, and desires. Healthy people are better

able to tap into and use their creative energy to lead productive, satisfying lives.

In addition to discussing the mind and overall well-being, this book explores natural medicine treatments for specific mental conditions. It covers the effects of stress on health—how it affects the mind and body by suppressing the immune system—and ways to cope with it in your daily life. The book also discusses the origins of anxiety disorders and depression, two of the most widespread mental disorders in contemporary society, and offers information about safe and effective natural treatments for overcoming them.

It is a sad fact that many people suffering from mental illness do not seek or receive adequate help for their problems, mostly because of a pervasive ignorance in our society. Illnesses of the mind seem to be shrouded in mystery and shame, almost as if they represent some weakness of character on the part of the victim. But what is important to realize and always bear in mind is that mental conditions are illnesses in the same way that heart disease and ulcers are illnesses. There are physiological bases for them, and sometimes they can be treated just as physical illnesses can be treated.

Illnesses of the mind such as anxiety and depression are, in fact, sometimes caused by physical malfunctions or chemical imbalances within the body. Environmental and psychological factors, such as stress or other emotional trauma, also play a role in triggering or perpetuating these imbalances in the body's biochemistry. Stress-related illness, anxiety, and depression in particular are extremely common in our society, and yet their symptoms are often ignored or misdiagnosed. Both doctors and patients need to be more aware of the symptoms of mental illness and how it can be treated. As a society, we need to educate ourselves about mental illness in order to dispel the ignorance and stigma attached to it. Only by doing this can we create a healthier environment for everyone.

Conventional medicine treats anxiety and depression with combinations of psychotherapy and drugs. Psychotherapies range in kind from psychoanalytic to behavioral, from individual to group formats, and from talk to action-oriented therapy. Psychotherapy, which will not harm but will most likely help a patient, is a viable natural medicine treatment that is discussed in more detail in Chapter 2.

Since the 1950s, when the first successful neuroleptics were marketed, pharmaceutical companies have forged ahead to discover and manufacture drugs to treat a host of mental disorders. Many of these drugs have proven highly effective, but they do come with a risk of causing numerous adverse side effects. Drugs are essential in treating many mental illnesses, such as severe depression, bipolar disorder, and schizophrenia. The danger lies in cases that do not necessarily warrant them. The tendency in conventional medicine as a whole is to prescribe the "magic bullet" that will relieve the patient's symptoms. But it is important to take into account the entire individual—job, lifestyle, habits, diet, and so on—to determine the root causes of illness. In the case of mild anxiety and depression, the causes often can be alleviated without the use of drugs simply by making adjustments in daily living. In such instances, the drugs would merely mask the symptoms without getting at the true underlying causes.

Most mental illnesses require some form of psychotherapy. While medication may be essential for certain individuals and illnesses, the natural treatments presented in this book are beneficial complements to conventional medicine. Oriental medicine, physical therapies, hydrotherapy, and exercise all play a vital role in reducing tension and stress. Homeopathic and herbal tonics can help restore balance to the body's biochemistry. Good nutrition, of course, is also a key to bolstering overall health.

This volume in The Dell Natural Medicine Library will help you gain a better understanding of the connection between the mind and the body. It explores the ways in which mental attitudes affect physical health and discusses alternative treatments for specific mental illnesses. When combined with conventional medicine, these natural therapies can help provide maximum healing and promote and maintain total well-being.

CHAPTER ONE

What Is Natural Medicine?

Acid rain . . . the disappearing ozone layer . . . smog . . . radiation . . . contaminated well water . . . It has become evident, from media reports as well as from personal experiences, that our increasing knowledge and technology can both help to advance society as well as wreak havoc on our lives. In a similar way, as the science of medicine has become more technical and has made great strides in treating many illnesses, it also has become more and more manipulative of and invasive to the human body. Unnecessary surgeries, excessive medication, life-support mechanisms . . . all of these alter the natural processes of health and illness, life and death. One cannot deny the value of surgery and medication in treating certain ailments and diseases, but it seems that we often lose sight of the body's power and ability, with the proper care and nurturing, to heal itself.

This notion of healing oneself is at the root of natural medicine philosophy. As more people witness the harmful effects of technology and the overuse of conventional modern medicine, they are turning to alternatives that are less invasive and disruptive of the body's natural processes. The new "health-consciousness craze" of the

1990s is all around us. People are striving to eat the right foods and maintain their proper weight; more people have made exercise a regular part of their daily routine; and some have discovered the benefits of relaxation and meditation, two elements that are particularly vital in our fast-paced, hectic lives.

You might grant that diet, exercise, and stress reduction are all well and good, yet doubt that they are a sufficient means of curing specific illnesses. How can riding the Lifecycle for twenty minutes three times a week possibly help chronic acid indigestion? The missing link is the mind: Proper care of your body helps create a healthy mind, and a balanced mind leads to a healthy body. They are interrelated; some believe they are one and the same. As a society, we are skeptical—we like to have things proven through testing and experimentation, and we like to see the facts. The brain and neurological system can be viewed as the physical embodiment of the mind, and this is true to the extent that scientists and doctors can measure and test these vital organs. The mind, however, is more than a mass of nerves, hormones, and electrical impulses. It represents an invisible, intangible, yet extremely powerful energy that, unfortunately, we often are too quick to dismiss.

Throughout history the mind has been viewed as something that must be mastered and controlled, otherwise one might "lose one's mind" or "go out of one's mind." An inability to control one's mind signified personal weakness to many people. It is useful, however, to think of the mind not as something to be controlled lest one go mad, but as energy to be harnessed and used to restore and maintain overall health. Indeed, this is the underlying philosophy of the practice of natural medicine.

Vis medicatrix naturae—the healing power of nature— this is the premise of natural medicine, which involves the use of an array of noninvasive, natural therapies to help restore balance to the body and thus help the system to heal itself. These therapies, which will be discussed individually in Chapter 2, include Oriental medicine, homeopathy, hydrotherapy, botanical medicine, physical medicine, psychotherapy, biofeedback, and nutrition. Natural medicine discourages the use of treatments that weaken the body's innate ability to heal itself, and although a person sometimes requires more than natural remedies, the natural medicine practitioner will always try to use the least invasive treatment possible.

Natural medicine functions from a holistic point of view; that is, your whole being is treated, rather than simply the part of your body that is sick. Natural medicine practitioners will take into consideration not only your obvious and immediate symptoms, but lifestyle, psychological factors, and other physical imbalances that may be present. They believe that illness affects the whole person —physically, emotionally, and mentally—and that imbalances within and among these three spheres will cause a person to exhibit symptoms of sickness. Natural medicine requires you to become involved in your own healing and to claim responsibility for your own health. Doctors have long been considered teachers of a certain kind, and natural medicine practitioners continue the tradition of educating their patients to become more aware of their own bodies, emotions, and minds and to help the self-healing process along.

Natural medicine strives for a balance between mind and body. If appropriate and necessary, various therapies can be used concurrently, or they can be used to supplement standard medical treatment if the case warrants it. The fact is that no one remedy or therapy—whether it is conventional or alternative—can work for everyone all of the time. The key is to explore your options and use the treatment that is most successful in treating your overall health and well-being.

Natural therapies are gaining popularity as people increasingly realize that conventional medicine cannot always offer all the answers or cures. According to a study published in the *New England Journal of Medicine* in January 1993, approximately one-third of all Americans used alternative medicine therapies in 1990, including relaxation techniques, massage, macrobiotic diets, spiritual healing, self-help groups, biofeedback, acupuncture, hypnosis, chiropractic, herbal medicine, and homeopathy. Patients spent $10.3 billion on alternative health care in 1990, and 90 percent of the treatments were sought by patients without the advice or suggestion of their regular physician.

The mainstream health-care industry, likewise, is changing to keep up with the growing demand for alternative medicine. The National Institutes of Health, at the urging of Congress, established an Office for the Study of Unconventional Medicine Practices and an Office of Alternative Medicine in 1992. Some conventional physicians have incorporated natural medicine philosophy and technique into their own practices. Insurance companies such as the American Western Life Insurance Company of California, the Mutual of Omaha Insurance Company, Blue

Cross of Washington and Alaska, and the New Jersey–based Prudential have extended coverage to include natural therapies. Clearly, natural medicine is becoming more popular as patients seek alternative treatments to those offered by Western medicine.

DIFFERENCES BETWEEN CONVENTIONAL AND ALTERNATIVE MEDICINE

Standard, conventional, or orthodox medicine, also called *allopathy,* defines health as the absence of disease. This definition is based on a negative. In contrast, holistic medicine concurs with the definition of health used by the World Health Organization (WHO), which posits that it is a state of complete physical, mental, and social well-being.

The allopathic and holistic definitions of health differ greatly in regard to the diagnosis and treatment of illness. People who use conventional medicine usually do not seek treatment until they become ill; there is little emphasis on preventive treatment. Holistic medicine, in contrast, focuses on preventing illness and maintaining health. The best illustration of this approach is the fact that ancient Chinese doctors were paid only when their patients were healthy, not if they became ill.

Natural medicine, which follows a holistic approach, views illness and disease as an imbalance of the mind and body that is expressed on the physical, emotional, and mental levels of a person. Although allopathy does recognize that many physical symptoms have mental components (for example, emotional stress might promote an ulcer or chronic headaches), its approach is generally to suppress the symptoms, both physical and psychological. Natural medicine assesses the symptoms as a sign or reflection of a deeper instability within the person, and it tries to restore the physical and mental harmony that will then alleviate the symptoms.

Except for cases of severe physical trauma, most illness derives from a level of susceptibility that varies in different people. For instance, some people seem to catch every cold and flu virus that goes around, while others can go for years without so much as a sniffle or a cough. The level of susceptibility reflects the deepest state of one's being. Bacteria and germs, as well as carcinogens, allergens, and other toxins, are agents of illness waiting to prey on a susceptible host. These stimuli alone do not cause illness, but rather induce specific symptoms in susceptible persons. Certain bacteria are known to be associated with certain diseases, and there are bacteria living within our bodies all of the time. Hence, if bacteria were the cause of illness, we would probably be sick all of the time. Instead, illness occurs when an imbalance in the body allows the bacteria to reproduce uncontrollably. Natural medicine usually views this uncontrolled growth as a manifestation of disease, not a cause of it. Natural medicine practitioners believe that preventive medicine, or therapies designed to maintain and enhance health, can reduce people's susceptibility and therefore the frequency with which they become ill.

Because of the fundamental differences in the way that allopathic and alternative physicians define and view health and illness, they also assess and treat their patients in very different ways. Alternative practitioners believe that people can use the power and positive energy of their minds to defend themselves against disease. Symptoms, therefore, are not caused by illness, but reflect the body's best attempt to heal itself. Since allopathic doctors believe that symptoms are caused by disease, they also believe that alleviating the symptoms will foster cure. In contrast, the natural medicine practitioner will claim that suppressing symptoms fails to address the underlying cause of illness and, in fact, can drive the illness deeper into the body, causing more profound symptoms to develop.

For example, if a child has a fever, an allopathic doctor might prescribe acetaminophen. Although this can help to bring the fever down, it is not curing the illness, which must run its course. An alternative practitioner, on the other hand, would consider the fever to be an indication that the body is fighting the illness. A high temperature makes the body unsuitable for bacteria to grow, and so it is the body's natural defense against the infection. Of course, an excessively high fever can be dangerous and should be treated so as to reduce it.

The difference between allopathic and natural treatments also can be seen in relation to the common cold. An allopathic doctor might suggest using an antihistamine to dry up a runny nose. However, natural medicine believes that the flow of mucus, and indeed all bodily secretions, is significant to the healing process, as it rids the body of toxic substances. If you are the kind of person who likes the quick remedy—that magic syrup or pill—and does not want to endure the discomforts of illness in the recovery process, you will have to assess whether natural medicine is appropriate for you. All of the alternative therapies discussed in this book require that your mind be open to their philosophies and that you become an active participant in your own recovery and health promotion.

In allopathy, diagnostic testing is vital in order for the doctor to name and categorize the disease and to treat it. Often these tests are done routinely, sometimes for the purpose of protecting the doctor rather than actually to help the patient. Some diagnostic tests, such as excessive X rays, or the use of powerful drugs can even cause sickness, referred to as iatrogenic illness, meaning "doctor-caused."

Although modern holistic doctors might use some standard diagnostic tests, they are more concerned with the individual's life circumstances. When you visit an alternative practitioner for the first time, he or she will consult at length with you, or "take the case," as it is called. During this initial visit, which can last more than an hour, the doctor will interview you, making notes about your verbal and nonverbal communication. The practitioner will be careful not to compare you with another patient, as each individual is unique. The doctor will record his or her observations of you as well as your complaints and concerns and will most likely ask questions to better individualize the case. If you are seeking help for an acute illness, the doctor probably will focus on symptoms and feelings that have changed since you became ill. If you are complaining of a chronic ailment, the doctor will want to know as much as possible about your life and history. Conventional diagnostic testing can be useful in certain cases, but the alternative doctor's practice of "taking the case" allows him or her to get at the deeper source of your problem, rather than just treating your symptoms.

Natural medicine operates on Hippocrates' theory of *primum non nocere,* or "first do no harm." The goal is to treat illness with noninvasive, harmless remedies that invoke the body's innate healing powers. Natural medicine involves a comprehensive view of health, illness, treatment, and cure that meets the need of each individual person and helps to restore and maintain balance of the body and mind.

In some cases, natural treatment can suffice to cure an illness, but other times allopathic treatments are required. If this is the case, alternative treatments can still be used to enhance the effectiveness of allopathic medicine, providing maximum healing for the individual. Healthy individuals also can pursue natural medicine regimens to maintain and enhance their physical, emotional, and mental well-being.

HISTORY OF NATURAL MEDICINE IN THE WEST

The word *naturopathy* was not used until the late nineteenth century, although its philosophy originated with Hippocrates, whose school of medicine existed around 400 B.C. Earlier people believed that disease was caused by supernatural powers. Hippocrates devised the theory that everything natural had a rational basis and that the causes of disease could be found in natural elements, such as air, water, or food. He also believed in *vis medicatrix naturae,* or the healing power of nature, and that the body had its own ability to heal itself.

The years from 1780 to 1850 marked the Age of Heroic Medicine. During this time, "heroic" treatments, such as bleeding, intestinal purgings, and blistering of the skin, were used to cure patients of their ills. These treatments were painful and harmful, and they often made patients worse, or even induced death. It was believed that bleeding, accomplished by lancing a vein or using leeches, removed impurities from the body. Intestinal purgings were performed by using mercuric chloride, which today we know causes severe metal poisoning; vomiting was induced by using other poisonous substances. The Age of Heroic Medicine was male-dominated and elitist, excluding women and nonconventional doctors. Some physicians who opposed heroic medicine practiced alternatives such as herbalism.

In 1810, a German doctor named Samuel Hahnemann (1755–1843) became disenchanted with the standard medicine of his day and began the practice of homeopathy. *Homeopathy* is derived from two Greek roots meaning "similar" and "disease, suffering." It is a philosophy of health and cure that is based on the principle that like cures like. That is, natural substances that produce particular symptoms in a healthy person can cure a sick person with those same symptoms.

Hahnemann did not actually originate the philosophy that like cures like; Hippocrates and others also had explored this concept previously. However, he did develop the theory into a viable alternative medical practice, homeopathy, which is discussed in greater detail in Chapter 2.

When Hahnemann died at the age of eighty-eight in 1843, he had many followers in Europe. The first homeopathic doctor came to the United States in 1828. In 1836, the Hahnemann Medical College opened in Philadelphia, and the first national medical society, the American Institute of Homeopathy, was established in 1844. As people began to react against heroic medical practices and politics, the Popular Health Movement was formed. It called for the repeal of all medical licensing laws, which was achieved by the end of the 1840s. This allowed physicians to practice whatever form of medicine they believed in. It was in this atmosphere that homeopathy flourished in the United States and set the stage for other alternative medicines, such as naturopathy, to take root.

Realizing that they were losing their foothold, the allopaths organized the American Medical Association (AMA) in 1846. While attacking homeopathy, they tried to give allopathy a more positive definition by claiming the word was based on German roots meaning "all therapies." Allopathy thus began to allow that a variety of remedies could be effective in treating a disease. The AMA required state medical societies to expel homeopaths and alternative healers, and in the 1860s, charges often were brought against allopaths who associated with these doctors. Allopaths began to wrest control of city hospitals and boards of health, and they succeeded in reestablishing licensing laws in all states. As the Popular Health Movement dissolved, alternative healers virtually were driven out of practice and denied any political influence.

By the 1880s, the homeopathic movement was being destroyed not only by the AMA but by its own internal philosophical divisions. Two groups of homeopaths emerged: those who were pure homeopaths, called Hahnemannians, and a larger, more modern group that included allopathic practices in their work and that wanted to work with allopathic doctors rather than against them.

Dr. John Scheel of New York City coined the word *naturopathy* in 1895 to connote "nature cure." The earliest forms of natural treatments and preventions included good hygiene and hydrotherapy. Naturopathy began to be pursued in full force in the United States in 1902 by Benedict Lust, who had emigrated from Germany in 1892. He had grown dissatisfied with conventional medicine and was intrigued by the European health spas, especially their treatment involving water cures and fasts. By the end of the nineteenth century, water cure was recognized as a vital healing therapy and referred to by the term *hydrotherapy.*

Lust intended to practice and teach hydrotherapy in the United States. Soon, however, his followers broadened their practices and healing philosophy to include an array of modalities, such as nutritional therapy, herbal medicine, homeopathy, spinal manipulation, exercise, hydrotherapy, electrotherapy, and stress management. Lust believed that in order to achieve good health, people should eliminate excessive consumption of toxic substances (such as caffeine, drugs, and alcohol), exercise, strive for a good mental attitude, and amend their lifestyles to include natural remedies such as fasting, proper diet, hydrotherapy, mud baths, chiropractic, and the like. He opened the American School of Naturopathy in New York City, which graduated its first class in 1902.

Natural medicine became very popular in the United States in the early twentieth century until the mid-1930s. At that point, conventional medicine again began to rise to prominence and popularity because of several factors.

First, the chemical and drug industries, which benefit more economically from allopathic than natural medicine, financially supported foundations that subsidized conventional medical schools. Second, orthodox medicine began to use less harmful treatments, and advances in health-care technology, particularly in surgery, convinced the public that conventional medicine was superior to natural medicine. The orthodox medical arena again began passing legislation that either limited or prohibited alternative health-care systems from flourishing.

Within the past two decades, since the 1970s, natural medicine has begun to take hold again. Realizing that allopathic medicine may not have all of the answers or cures for their ills, people are seeking alternative treatments. As people begin to recognize the devastating contaminating effects of some technology on air, water, and food, they are beginning to take action against such harmful practices. Finally, as the connection between the mind and body becomes ever more apparent, people are willing to make major lifestyle changes in order to protect and maintain their sense of physical and emotional balance. This is what natural medicine is all about and it is why more and more people are realizing the long-term benefits of alternative medical treatments.

LOCATING A NATURAL MEDICINE PRACTITIONER

One of the best ways to find a good alternative practitioner is to be referred by one of his or her patients, though you might not be fortunate enough to find one in this way. At the end of this book is a list of Natural Medicine Resources. Contact the listed organizations. Often they can make referrals to practitioners in your area, or they may have membership directories available.

When consulting a practitioner, interview him or her to learn as much as you can about the person and his or her practice. As a result of the interview, you will feel more comfortable seeking help from this person if you decide to do so, and that level of trust and comfort will facilitate a beneficial outcome for your treatment. The American Holistic Medical Association can send you a publication, *How to Choose a Holistic Health Practitioner.* The organization's address is listed in the Natural Medicine Resources section. Following are some questions to ask a practitioner you interview:

- What schools did you attend and what is the extent of your training?
- What licenses or certificates do you hold?
- How long have you been in practice?
- What are your diagnostic and treatment procedures?
- What are the fees involved? What is the length of treatment or number of sessions proposed?
- Have you written any articles or books? (If so, they may be worth reading.)

CHAPTER TWO

Natural Therapies:
An Overview

ORIENTAL MEDICINE

Oriental medicine defines health not as an absence of disease, as in Western medicine, but as a total state of well-being. It requires that the body be free from physical pain, but also encompasses the totality of the individual's thoughts, emotions, and beliefs. Health, in Eastern philosophy, is a state of mind and a way of life. Illness results from going against the natural laws of Heaven and Earth.

Oriental medicine began at least three thousand years ago, and has developed progressively as a science since approximately A.D. 200. It continues to flourish in the Eastern countries today, and many aspects of Oriental medicine are beginning to gain popularity as alternative treatments in the West. Oriental medicine involves several healing therapies, including acupuncture, herbs, nutrition, exercise (such as tai chi chuan and other martial arts), massage, and manipulation.

Taoism, Confucianism, and Buddhism are the underlying philosophies of Chinese medicine. According to Taoism, health reflects a harmony in Heaven, which is achieved through the balance of external and internal forces. A unity exists within the diversity of nature—a universal energy that exists in all things. This energy, called *chi,* is very difficult to describe. It has been explained as matter on the verge of becoming energy, while at the same time it is also energy on the verge of becoming matter. Everything in the universe is a result of the never-ending condensation of *chi* into matter and dispersion of *chi* into energy. In terms of Chinese medicine, *chi* needs to be understood in two ways. First, it nourishes the mind and body and has been described as the life force. Second, *chi* is produced by and indicates the function of the various *zang/fu,* or "spheres of function." *Zang/fu* refers not to a specific organ, such as the liver, but to the totality of body functions associated with the liver. Stomach *chi,* therefore, refers to various stomach functions, such as the transportation of food essences. The Chinese believe that *chi* flows throughout the human body. Health reflects a free flow of *chi,* but if the energy is imbalanced —if there is a blockage, an excess, or a deficiency of *chi* in specific body parts or organs—disease and illness occur.

Taoism also recognizes two opposite yet complementary qualities to all aspects of physical being. The philosophy derives from the notion that the universe was originally a ball of *chi* surrounded by chaos. When this mass of energy finally settled, it divided into the two opposing yet complementary qualities called *yin* and *yang.* Yin represents qualities that are negative, contractive, dark, small, of the right side, interior, of the nature of Earth. Yang, in contrast, is positive, expansive, light, big, of the left side, surface, of the nature of Heaven. All objects, animals, peoples, times, and places are a combination of yin and yang. It is believed that people are born with perfect yin and yang balance that is later thrown off kilter. Chinese doctors designate certain organs as being either of yin or yang qualities, and so are the foods and medicinal herbs that would be used to treat ailments of these organs.

Practitioners of Chinese medicine and philosophers believe in a dynamic cycle of evolution known as the five-element theory. All things are classified according to the five elements of wood, fire, earth, metal, and water. The body's organs are also characterized by the five elements; for example, the spleen and stomach are of the earth, and the lung and large intestine are of metal. These five elements are in a state of constant change and interact with one another. Doctors believe that organs affect other organs according to the elements. For instance, wood generates fire; therefore, the activity of the liver, which is characterized by wood, generates the activity of the heart, which is a fire organ. The relationships between the elements show doctors the direction in which *chi* flows within the body.

Just as the Chinese views about health differ from Western notions, so do their ideas about human anatomy. Chinese doctors identify twelve organs, or the *zang/fu,* which do not correspond directly to organs as we know them. Remember that *zang/fu* refers not to a specific organ, but to all of the body functions associated with that organ. This way of looking at the body probably evolved because ancient Chinese tradition prohibited the opening of corpses. Therefore, rather than developing a more detailed, concrete knowledge of anatomy, scientists and doctors focused on body functions instead of specific organs. The result is a more holistic understanding of function that embraces physical, mental, and emotional aspects.

Chinese medicine requires that the flow of *chi* in the body be influenced or moved, either by the practitioner or by the patient, so as to restore its balance. The flow of *chi* can be impeded by poor nutrition; lack of exercise; mental stress; fatigue; bad posture and breathing; pollution; physical growths such as tumors; or trauma, including those that result in scar tissue. A deficiency in *chi* can cause fatigue, depression, and various physical ailments. Excess *chi* might be responsible for hypertension, migraine headaches, or some types of arthritis. If the natural flow of *chi* through the body is altered in any way, a host of ailments could occur.

Chi flows through the body in fourteen pathways called meridians. The geography of the human body, as viewed by Eastern doctors, is based on these pathways as well as the *zang/fu* (organs) and bowels, and is very different from Western concepts of anatomy and physiology. Twelve of the meridians pass through a major organ and are linked to other meridians, so that all body parts have access to *chi*.

Practitioners of Oriental medicine examine and diagnose their patients in a way that is quite different from the quick, routine examinations and consultations patients in the West are accustomed to. There is careful questioning and observation of the patient, as well as monitoring of the patient's pulse. This is not pulse-checking as we know it, however. Rather, it is a fine art of detecting several layers of pulses in order to determine which body spheres are suffering. The doctor will take a pulse using the first three fingers of his or her hand, checking the patient's wrists with both light and firm pressure. The doctor will also identify pulses under each finger at both pressure levels—a total of six pulses for each wrist. Each pulse correlates with a specific body function sphere.

Acupuncture

One of the major Oriental healing arts is acupuncture, which involves the insertion of needles at specific points on the body. These special points are located along the various meridians, twelve of which correspond to a particular organ. It is indeed an art as well as a science to be able to locate the precise point at which a needle should be inserted. If it is not placed in the right position, the procedure will not have the desired effect. The purpose of acupuncture is to move or restore the flow of *chi* through the insertion of the needles along the meridians relevant to the illness.

The needles are inserted quickly and left in place for several minutes. Sometimes the doctor will just pierce the skin, while other times the needle will be inserted up to an inch deep. The doctor might twirl the needle to increase stimulation. Another process of stimulating the acupuncture points is called *moxabustion.* In one method of moxabustion, the needles' heads are wrapped with dry *moxa* (Chinese wormwood) and burned. The needle conducts the heat into the acupuncture point. In yet another process, called electroacupuncture, the doctor connects each needle to a small machine that stimulates the needles with a low electrical pulse.

To those people raised with Western medical treatments, acupuncture is often viewed as a superstitious practice. The thought of having needles inserted into various regions of the body, even places as delicate as the face, can make even the staunchest Westerner squeamish. Those who have experienced acupuncture, however, claim that it is a painless, effective treatment for many illnesses. An acupuncture patient probably will feel a slight sensation when the needles are inserted. As the acupuncture works, the patient also might feel the presence of *chi* at the sites of the needles or the movement of *chi* in the body.

All this discussion about *chi* and influencing its movement through the body may be difficult for you to accept. Western scientists and doctors have devised several theories to explain why acupuncture works, especially when it is used to alleviate pain. One theory is based on the fact that the body produces endorphins and enkephalins, natural painkilling chemicals that also can help allergies and depression and can facilitate healing. Stimulating acupuncture points increases the body's production of endorphins and enkephalins. Another theory to explain acupuncture is that it has a placebo effect if the patient truly believes that it will help. Still another is based on the fact that some scientists and doctors feel that our vital energy is not *chi,* as the Chinese know it, but rather electricity. Acupuncture affects the way electricity travels along the meridians. Kirlian photography, which illustrates bioelectricity, provides evidence that this is a viable theory. The picture of a hand before and after acupuncture reveals an increased flow of electricity after the treatment. Finally, the gate theory of pain also is used to explain acupuncture. According to this theory, the body contains neuropathway "gates" along the spinal cord leading to the brain. Acupuncture closes the gates so that messages of pain do not reach the brain.

From a Chinese medicine point of view, acupuncture works as a result of regulating the flow of *chi* and blood. There is a Chinese expression, "There is no pain if there is free flow; if there is pain, there is no free flow."

Acupuncture has been shown to be an effective analgesic and has even been used instead of anesthetics during surgery. The stimulation of the acupuncture points in order to produce an analgesic effect causes the brain to release endorphins, which are the body's natural painkilling chemicals. Although Chinese doctors might use anesthetics during an operation, using acupuncture as an analgesic necessitates using only a fraction of the dose that a surgical patient in the West would receive. This is especially important for people who are sensitive to painkillers and anesthesia, as acupuncture is a harmless, safe way to treat pain.

Acupuncture can be an effective treatment for both terminal and nonterminal illnesses. A therapy that can be used alone or in combination with another treatment, it is also useful in dealing with the side effects of conventional medicine.

If you are considering acupuncture as a healing therapy, try to get a referral from an acupuncture society or school, from the pain clinic at your local hospital, or from someone who has experienced the treatment firsthand. Investigate the training and experience of the doctor until you are satisfied with his or her qualifications. Licensing varies by state: Some license independent practitioners, while others restrict practice to medical doctors (those with an M.D. degree) or allow acupuncturists to work only under such a doctor's supervision. Contact the American Association of Acupuncture and Oriental Medicine, the National Commission for the Certification of Acupuncturists, or the National Accreditation Commission for Schools and Colleges of Acupuncture and Oriental Medicine (see the Natural Medicine Resources section) for information regarding licensing requirements in your state and for more information about acupuncture.

Visits to an acupuncturist range in cost from $35 to $75. Some insurance companies do cover the cost of acupuncture, but many still do not, and some will cover only those treatments recommended by a conventional doctor. Be sure to check your policy regarding your coverage for acupuncture.

When you visit an acupuncturist, make sure that the doctor uses either presterilized disposable needles or an autoclave, which is a sterilizing machine. An autoclave is the only effective way to sterilize needles and other medical or dental instruments sufficiently.

To many people in the West, acupuncture is a strange procedure, of which they are skeptical. It is an art and a science that has been practiced for thousands of years, however, and its effects and benefits are often not acknowledged by orthodox Western medicine.

Acupressure

Acupressure is a therapy that is similar to acupuncture in that it uses the same geography of meridians and acupuncture (or acupressure) points. Instead of using needles, however, hands or feet gently pressure the appropriate points. Acupressure relaxes tense muscles, improves blood circulation, and stimulates the body's ability to heal itself.

Acupressure, which predates acupuncture, was developed approximately five thousand years ago by the Chinese. They discovered that pressing certain points on the body not only relieved localized pain, but could affect other parts of the body and internal organs as well. Acupressure was increasingly disregarded, however, as the Chinese began to use needles to stimulate the acupressure points.

Acupressure points are illustrated on pages 277–80 at the back of the book. The descriptions of treatments for various conditions will refer to these diagrams and name the corresponding numbers that are relevant to use. For example, in treating migraine headaches, the text will read: "GB 20, located below the base of the skull in the hollows between the vertical neck muscles." Once you locate the point on yourself or the person you are treating, apply firm and steady pressure. It will take practice and experimentation to find the points and pressure that work for you.

Acupressure is not intended to cure serious illness or replace orthodox medical treatments for those illnesses. It can, however, increase relaxation, improve circulation, and ease pain, thereby maximizing health. Since it utilizes the same points as in acupuncture, specific *chi* or blood regulating or nourishing benefits associated with the points can be realized. It is an inexpensive and simple therapy to learn and one that, if practiced correctly, is entirely safe. Here are some tips to bear in mind when administering acupressure to yourself or others:

• Use only gentle pressure; it should not cause any pain.

- Since there are a number of acupoints that are forbidden during pregnancy, you should work on a pregnant woman only under the instruction of a qualified acupuncture or acupressure practitioner.
- Do not use acupressure on someone who is taking drugs or alcohol.
- Do not administer acupressure immediately after eating.
- It is best for the patient to sit or lie down, as he or she may feel drowsy during a procedure.

Movement and Meditation

Advocates of Oriental medicine also believe that you can heal yourself through the dedicated practice of different kinds of movement and meditation.

The martial arts are different forms of exercise that require and develop supreme control, discipline, and strength in the individual. A gentle martial art, tai chi chuan, can help a person develop inner strength and control. The Chinese believe that movement is essential for the human body. Tai chi chuan involves slow, deliberate movements, a sense of communion with nature, and concentration on finding one's *chi*. The philosophy is that if one can locate one's *chi* and learn how to use it, one can maintain good health. Some martial arts schools offer classes in tai chi chuan, and it is an exercise that requires many years of dedicated practice to develop fully.

Another form of meditation, called chi-gong, is also used to find one's *chi*. Chinese doctors believe that a ball of *chi* is located in the abdominal or pelvic region, and through meditation people can learn to move their *chi* to the appropriate areas of their body. The idea, again, is to learn to influence the flow of *chi* so as to maintain its balance in the body.

Whether you are working with a doctor or trying to heal yourself, all Oriental medicine seems to require willing and dedicated participation on your part. Oriental medicine has been practiced for thousands of years, and it is effective. Of course, as with any healing treatment, not all forms will work in every case or all of the time. Oriental medicine does seem to substantiate, however, the connection of the mental and physical. This belief is inherent in the Eastern philosophy of health, and it is utilized to treat illness and to maximize health.

HOMEOPATHY

Homeopathy is a system of health care and treatment that was developed in the 1800s by Dr. Samuel Hahnemann. The philosophy of homeopathy is holistic, viewing the individual as a totality of interdependent parts and working from the notion that the mental and physical realms are inseparable. Hahnemann believed that orthodox medicine was a system of "contraries," meaning that doctors treated the symptoms of an illness by using drugs that oppose, or suppress, them. He began to call conventional medicine *allopathic,* meaning "different" and "disease, suffering." Hahnemann recognized that removing or masking symptoms did not treat the underlying cause of the illness, which could, in effect, develop into a more serious condition.

In homeopathy, symptoms are seen as a healthy response of the body's defense mechanism. The vital force, or vital energy, acts to keep the body in balance. When the body is threatened by some harmful external influence, the vital force (or defense mechanism) produces symptoms in its struggle against the harmful agent. Therefore, to a homeopathic doctor, fever is a sign that the body is fighting illness. A cough, which an allopathic doctor would try to suppress with medication, is seen by the homeopath as the natural way to expel mucus from the body. Bear in mind that this does not mean you must suffer with coughing all day long. You can use herbal cough drops and drink teas with honey, for example, to soothe your throat. However, if you are not willing to endure some discomfort during your sickness, you should reassess whether natural medicine treatments are appropriate for you.

Believing that drug prescriptions for specific illnesses often were based on an inadequate understanding of the drugs and their effects, Hahnemann began to test, or "prove," drugs on healthy women and men, including himself, to determine their effects. He tested remedies on people rather than animals because he knew that people usually react differently than animals do. This human testing is possible because the homeopathic remedies are nontoxic. In more than two hundred years of using the homeopathic formulations, there has been no reported case of a permanent adverse reaction.

In his provings, Hahnemann discovered that each remedy induced particular symptoms in a healthy person. When that remedy was given to a sick person exhibiting those same symptoms, it helped cure the person. Based on this notion that like cures like, Hahnemann formulated the Law of Similars. It states that a substance causing certain symptoms in a healthy person can cure a sick person with the same symptoms. The theory behind the Law of Similars is that the body enlists its own energies to heal itself and defend against illness. If a substance that causes a similar response in terms of similar symptoms is administered, the body steps up its fight against it, thereby promoting cure.

In an attempt to lessen the initial aggravating effects that remedies sometimes had on patients, Hahnemann administered very small dosages. Ironically, he discovered that the smaller the dose, the more powerful the effect. This led him to develop the Law of Infinitesimals, which states that the smaller the dose, the more effective it is in stimulating the body to respond against the illness.

In order to prepare smaller and smaller doses, Hahnemann would put a substance through a series of dilutions. He would begin with the original substance, putting one part in nine parts of an 87 percent solution of alcohol and distilled water. He then subjected to *succussion,* or vigorously agitated, the vial by striking it one hundred times against a leather pad. Hahnemann believed that subjecting the substance to succussion activated the therapeutic potential of it. This first step yields a one-in-ten dilution, also indicated as a "1× dilution." Hahnemann would then take one part of this 1× dilution and put it in nine parts of diluent, subjecting it to succussion to yield a 2× dilution. This process, referred to as the Law of Potentization, could continue indefinitely, producing increasingly potent dosages.

Hahnemann believed in administering one homeopathic remedy at a time in order to establish its effects. He treated all patients as whole people, taking their symptoms as part of their whole being rather than treating them separately, and apart from the rest of the person. This method differs from orthodox medicine in which specialists treat specific illnesses and body parts, and patients often take many drugs simultaneously.

Homeopathy views health as a state of freedom and well-being on three interdependent levels: physical, emotional, and mental. The most serious symptoms usually affect the deeper parts of a person; therefore, it is most important to treat the mental state, then the emotional, and finally the physical. This is in keeping with the holistic view of natural medicine, which treats the entire person—physically and mentally. In other words, a homeopath would say that it is not enough to treat you for migraine headaches, because if the stressors producing the migraines are not addressed, the migraines will recur or other symptoms could develop.

The German homeopath Constantine Hering, who emigrated to the United States in the 1830s, recorded the changes in posttreatment symptoms. Based on his findings that healing occurs from the inside out, he laid the groundwork for Hering's Law of Cure, which is recognized not only by homeopaths but by acupuncturists and psychotherapists as well.

Hering's Law states that cure occurs from within outward, from the most vital to the least important organs. The body deals with the most significant aspect of the condition first, shifting during treatment to the next most important aspect, and so on. For instance, healing is believed to be in progress—from the inside out—if your chest pains subside but a skin rash develops. During homeopathic treatment, your condition can change so that the same or other remedies may be needed to facilitate the entire process of cure.

Hering's Law further states that symptoms will appear and disappear in the reverse order in which they originally appeared. The patient may also reexperience symptoms from a past condition. According to Hering, healing often begins with the upper body parts and descends. Therefore, if chronic headaches subside but stiff fingers are felt, the homeopath might believe that healing is taking place, and gradually the fingers should return to normal. At times, healing may not follow the traditional pattern of Hering's Law, but as long as the patient feels stronger and is improved overall, it is safe to assume that the treatment is working.

Based on the order "first, do no harm," homeopathy is a safe and effective system of treating many common acute and chronic ailments. For a temporary, minor, self-limited illness or injury, you probably can treat yourself with homeopathic remedies after consulting with your doctor. You can obtain remedies from homeopathic pharmacists, or even from some drugstores or health-food stores. For a more chronic, persistent illness, you should consult a qualified homeopathic practitioner. Professional homeopathic medical doctors graduate from conventional four-year medical schools with a Doctor of Medicine (M.D.) degree and often complete postgraduate training in homeopathy to learn this holistic specialty. Homeopathic schools can be found worldwide, but to master the art and science of the system, physicians often learn from experienced homeopathic doctors. The fees charged by homeopaths vary, as does insurance coverage. Some states and insurance companies honor homeopathic treatment and some do not, and some will cover it only if it is performed by a licensed medical doctor.

HYDROTHERAPY

Sometimes the most obvious and simplest remedies are the ones most often overlooked. Consider water—it composes two thirds of our bodies and covers four fifths of the earth's surface. Human beings can survive for weeks without food but only a few days without water. How can an element so common and abundant possibly be useful in healing?

The use that probably comes to mind first is the practice of swimming as physical therapy or bathing in a whirlpool to soothe sore muscles. But water has other healthful benefits as well, and in its various forms it can even be used to treat injuries and illnesses. It can work on the whole body, as in a bath, or on one area, as in the use of a compress. Water benefits the entire body by reenergizing it. Using a water therapy on one body part can also affect another beneficially, such as the use of a hot footbath to aid decongestion. Every organ and cell requires water, which helps nourish, detoxify, and maintain the right temperature of the body.

One of the earliest records of the therapeutic use of water dates back to the Greek god of medicine known as Aesculapius. At his temples, bathing and massage were used as a form of cure. Hippocrates also used water therapeutically. He advocated drinking water to alleviate fever, and he believed that baths could fight sickness. The Greek doctor Galen, who wrote Rome's outstanding medical text, also believed baths, both hot and cold, had beneficial effects, as did the Greek medical writer Celsus. Of course, this is true, because, in fact, one of the major reasons that health has increased over the ages is that sanitation and hygiene have improved.

In the eighteenth century, German, English, and Italian clergy revived the therapeutic use of water. In 1797, a Scottish doctor, James Currie, wrote a book called *Medical Reports on the Effects of Water, Cold and Warm, as a Remedy in Fever and Febrile Diseases.* In the early nineteenth century, Vincent Preissnitz, a Silesian farmer, reinvented water therapy using methods such as dousings, showers, immersions, and single and double compresses. His procedures spread to England, Germany, and Scandinavia, as well as the United States.

Later in the nineteenth century, Sebastian Kniepp adapted Preissnitz's techniques into his own theories of hydrotherapy. Kniepp, born in Bavaria in 1821, was a frail and sickly person. After reading a pamphlet about water cures, he decided to plunge into an icy cold river in the middle of winter with the hope that it would cure his ailments. Kniepp jumped into the river every day, and although it might seem absurd, he claimed that over time he became physically stronger. Along with Preissnitz's techniques, Kniepp claimed that walking in cold water or on wet grass was therapeutic.

Hydrotherapy is based on the law of action and reaction. If the skin is heated, either by a hot bath or compress, blood is immediately drawn to the surface and then returns to the deeper blood vessels. Likewise, cold water will drive blood away from the surface, but will cause a secondary effect of warmth as the blood returns to the tissues and vessels from which it was pushed away. This concept of immediate action followed by a secondary and more lasting reaction is a basic principle of hydrotherapy.

The different forms and temperatures of water have different physical and chemical effects on the body. Cold water is essentially restorative and reenergizing. It can reduce fever, act as a diuretic and anesthetic, alleviate pain, help relieve constipation, and eliminate toxins from the body. Ice and ice water can relieve the pain of burns, help control bleeding, and reduce swelling from injury. Warm water, in contrast, has a relaxing effect. Hot baths induce perspiration, which is essential in eliminating toxins from the body. Hot compresses and baths can reduce pain and inflammation, although cold water should be used for inflammation due to injury. This is important because hot water increases blood flow and would thereby increase inflammation in an injury. Alternating hot and cold baths can help increase circulation. Steam is a form of hydrotherapy that opens pores, increases perspiration, and sometimes alleviates chest congestion. Humidifying air is good for those who suffer from sinus conditions and airborne allergies.

Water has therapeutic uses when used internally or externally, at varying degrees of temperatures and pressures, and in its three forms: ice, liquid, or steam. Ice can be used as an anesthetic to chill the skin and dull pain. Boiling water is an antiseptic that can cleanse food and clothing. Hot compresses placed on the abdomen and herbal teas can work as antispasmodics to relieve cramps. If you need a diuretic, try drinking ice water or herbal tea or applying a hot, moist compress on your lower back; these all affect the kidneys to increase urine production. Colon irrigation, enemas, genital irrigation, the drinking of water, the taking of a sauna or hot baths all help to eliminate toxins. Drinking an emetic, such as salt water, can induce vomiting in order to expel certain poisonous substances. Finally, hot or cold baths or showers, whirlpools, and salt baths have a stimulating effect, while warm showers or herbal baths can act as a sedative.

Many different types of water application are used in hydrotherapy. Local heat can be achieved with a moist, hot compress or hot-water bottle; local cold requires a cold compress, frozen bandage, or ice pack or bag. A cold double compress is a cold compress covered with a dry cloth, such as wool or flannel, which creates internal heat. A pack is a larger form of the double compress, or it can be a clay, mustard, or flaxseed poultice. Alcohol, water, or witch hazel can be used in sponging, and you can achieve tonic friction by rubbing with a sponge or washcloth. Therapeutic showers can alternate between hot and cold, and the pressure of the shower can vary. Steam is therapeutic too, from a sauna, vaporizer, or humidifier.

One of the most common and most appreciated hydrotherapy techniques is the bath, a total immersion of either the body or a part of the body, such as hands, feet, arms, eyes, or fingers. Depending on the ailment you wish to treat, baths can be cold, tepid, or hot, can be long or short in duration, and can involve massage using a sponge, bath mitten, or loofah brush to create tonic friction. Baths can consist of plain water or contain salts, herbs, oatmeal, or mud. Following is a list of bath additives and their therapeutic benefits:

Apple cider vinegar: Fights fatigue; relieves sunburn and itchy skin.

Borax/cornstarch/bicarbonate of soda: Good antiseptic.

Bran: Softens skin, and relieves itchiness.

Chamomile: Soothes skin and opens pores; helps to relieve insomnia and digestive problems.

Dead Sea salts: Restores body after injury.

Epsom salts: Increases perspiration, relaxes muscles, and helps to relieve catarrh.

Fennel/nettle: Helps to rid skin of impurities.

Ginger powder: Relaxes muscles, tones skin, and increases circulation. (Use in small amounts, as it is very powerful.)

Hayflower/oatstraw: Helps to rid skin of impurities.

Nutmeg: Increases perspiration.

Oatmeal: Good for skin problems, such as itchiness, hives, windburn, and sunburn.

Pine: Increases perspiration, softens skin, and relieves rashes.

Rosemary: Stimulates blood circulation.

Sage: Stimulates sweat glands.

Salt: Promotes a relaxing effect.

Sulfur: Good antiseptic and helps to rid skin of parasites; helps relieve acne.

It is easy and inexpensive to treat yourself to a wide variety of baths. Most of the listed herbs and preparations can be bought in drugstores, herbal pharmacies, health-food stores, or through catalogs. Remember to purchase them in small quantities since they lose their potency in approximately one year.

BOTANICAL MEDICINE

Botanical medicine, also referred to as herbalism, plant healing, physiomedicalism, medical herbalism, and phytotherapy, uses remedies made from plants called herbs. Whereas botanists define herbs as any plants that do not contain woody fibers, medicinal herbalists define them as any plant that has healing properties. Herbal remedies can also come from trees, ferns, seaweeds, or lichens, and herbalists will use whole plants, rather than isolating the principal active compounds from them. Whole plants contain proteins, enzymes, vitamins, minerals, and other trace elements that readily assimilate in the body. In fact, the three fatty acids essential for life—linoleic, linolenic, and arachidonic—are all found in plants. Botanical medicine is a safe and natural way to treat specific ailments and assist recuperation from illness in order to restore physiological balance.

The history of botanical medicine goes back through the ages, with "recipes" for herbal remedies being passed from generation to generation. Plants are natural agents of cure, and animals have an instinct for their curative powers. You've probably seen a dog nibble on grass. No, he doesn't think he's part goat—but he might have a bellyache and is eating the grass to aid his digestion. For centuries, Native Americans have chewed willow-tree bark to cure headaches. The bark contains salicylic acid, the active ingredient in aspirin.

Traditional herbal medicine originated in ancient times in India, China, and Egypt, with the earliest records appearing in Egypt and Assyria. Many of the plants listed in these and in Greek documents are still used today. Over time, herbalists have compiled classifications—descriptions of plants arranged according to their medicinal properties. Today, there are more than 750,000 plants in the world, and only a small percentage have been evaluated. The World Health Organization investigates and supports herbal medicine throughout the world in order to learn more about this natural method of healing.

Plants are used not only in botanical medicine but in allopathic medicine as well, and once served as the basis for nearly all drugs. In order to appreciate the benefits of botanical medicine, it is useful to look at how allopathy has used plants in preparing drugs.

Until the 1800s, most drugs were given by mouth in the form of ground leaves, roots, or flowers, or in teas, tinctures, or extracts. Doctors studied botany as a matter of course, and herbalists without medical training, particularly women, also flourished.

Prior to the 1800s, there was no standard clinical evidence on which doctors could base their selection of drugs for treatment. In 1803, a German pharmacist isolated morphine from opium, signifying the first time that a pure active principle had been obtained from a crude plant drug. With this pure form of morphine, doctors could give exact doses, knowing their effects. In the mid-nineteenth century, there was a push to isolate pure forms of active principles from medicinal plants. By 1870, caf-

feine had been isolated from coffee, nicotine from tobacco, and cocaine from coca.

These isolated compounds are generally more toxic
than the whole plants from which they are derived. Scientists and doctors believed it was better to treat patients
with the purified drug, and they disregarded other compounds in the plant. Herbalists, however, recognized that
the whole plant has a different effect from the isolated
substance since it contains many other vital ingredients
that interact to give an overall effect.

Besides using isolated principles, chemists also experiment with molecules to synthesize new drugs. Their goal
usually is to increase the potency and efficacy of the drug.
More potent drugs can be risky, however, given that doctors often prescribe numerous medications simultaneously. And some drugs are so potent as to be addictive.
Adverse drug reactions, or side effects, are the most common effects of iatrogenic (doctor-caused) illness.

Many commonly used drugs are derived from plants.
For instance, digitoxin comes from foxglove *(Digitalis
purpurea)* and is prescribed for heart failure; atropine is
from deadly nightshade *(Atropa belladonna)* and dilates
pupils; morphine comes from the opium poppy *(Papaver
somniferum)* and is a powerful painkiller.

Herbalists may use the root, rhizome, stem, leaf,
flower, seed, fruit, bark, wood, resin, or whole plant in
preparing an herbal medication. Familiar with the inter-
action of various plants with each other, herbalists usually
will use several plants or extracts in one preparation, since
they can sometimes be more effective when combined
than when used separately. Plants contain oils, alkaloids
(nitrogen compounds), tannins, resins, fats, carbohy-

drates, proteins, and enzymes that all contribute to their medicinal action. Each substance has a function and can support, control, or otherwise affect the other constituents. In using the whole plant, the herbalist will get the most gentle, safe, and effective benefit from the treatment.

Herbal remedies can be taken in the form of tablets, capsules, lotions, ointments, suppositories, inhalants, or teas and juices. For herbal drinks, the basic proportion is 1 ounce (25 grams) herbs to 1 pint (0.5 liter) liquid. Herb teas will keep for three days in a tightly covered container in the refrigerator. Following is a list of common terms referring to botanical medications:

Carminative: Relieves flatulence, colic.

Cholagogue: Stimulates release of bile from the gallbladder.

Decoction: Drink made from roots, bark, or berries simmered in boiling water and strained.

Demulcent: Soothing substance for the skin.

Emmenagogue: Stimulates menstruation.

Emollient: Used internally to soothe membranes or externally to soften skin.

Infusion: Boiling water is poured over leaves, flowers, or the whole plant (excluding seeds and berries).

Nervine: That which is calming.

Ointments: Applied externally; effective for skin conditions.

Poultice: Crushed plant and hot water mixed to produce a paste that is wrapped in a thin cloth and applied to the skin.

Pressed juice: Juice from fresh plants is rich in vitamins and minerals; can be used in tinctures or diluted in water.

Teas: Made from pouring boiling water over fermented leaves or stalks from one or more plants; fermentation produces tannin; premade teabags can be purchased.

Tinctures: One part herb in five parts of diluted alcohol.

Tisane: Add boiling water to fresh or dried plant, usually green leaves.

You can dry your own leaves by laying them on a wire rack in a warm, dry place for forty-eight hours; store in airtight glass containers. This should keep for one year. When preparing a tisane, use a separate pot from tea, as tannin will interfere with the tisane remedy.

Vulnerary: Used to treat and heal wounds.

An herbalist can give you information as to appropriate herbs used to treat various symptoms. A consultation with an herbalist is similar to one with other natural healers. The herbalist will check your heart and pulse, physical symptoms, and perhaps perform some laboratory tests, such as blood and urine analyses. More important, the herbal practitioner will spend quite some time observing, talking, questioning, and listening to you in order to determine the imbalance and disharmony of your body and life.

If you find a satisfactory course of treatment with a particular herbalist, it is good to stay with that person so as not to disrupt the healing process. Sometimes symptoms are aggravated before healing occurs, and some people and certain disorders take longer to heal than others. Patience and willing participation in your treatment is essential in order to maximize the benefits of botanical medicine. An herbal treatment, however, should only be undertaken in consultation with your physician.

PHYSICAL MEDICINE

Chiropractic

The word *chiropractic* means "treatment by the hands, or manipulation." It is a system of healing that was developed by David Daniel Palmer (1845–1913) in Iowa in 1895. Palmer believed that displacements of the spine caused pressure on nerves, which created pain or symptoms in other parts of the body.

Although chiropractic medicine subscribes to traditional concepts of anatomy and physiology, it differs from traditional medicine in that it is holistic, meaning it considers the patient as a whole, with an emphasis on body structure. Practitioners rely on X rays and standard orthopedic and neurological tests to diagnose problems, focusing on abnormalities of the spine. Treatment often involves direct thrust on specific vertebrae that are out of alignment, which helps to restore the flow of energy. Two terms that you will encounter in chiropractic are *adjustment* and *manipulation*. Adjustments involve dynamic thrusts (rapid, precise, and painless force) to a specific vertebra in order to remove any interference with nerves. It is not only the adjustment itself that is important, but the body's healing reaction to it. Manipulations are more general reorderings of bones to realign joints and increase the patient's range of motion.

Chiropractic is helpful in treating many conditions, including back pain and musculoskeletal disorders as well as certain systemic illnesses, such as asthma, migraines, and digestive problems. These systemic disorders, however, can be helped only if there is evidence of a structural and neurological involvement. Chiropractic treatment must be administered by a qualified and licensed professional, and it usually involves multiple visits in order to maintain proper spinal alignment. Initial visits can run from $50 to $150, with routine visits priced at approximately $50, and most insurance companies do provide coverage for this treatment. Chiropractors usually undergo at least two years of college plus an additional four years of professional education, and they must pass state and national licensing examinations.

Massage

The word *massage* derives from both the Greek *masso* ("knead") and the Arabic *mass* ("press gently"). It is a form of physical medicine that is completely harmless, comfortable, and relaxing. While a massage can be given by anyone, a trained massage therapist often seems to have a magic touch.

Massage works on the soft tissues, muscles, and ligaments of the body. It stimulates circulation and the function of the nervous system and helps to lower blood pressure. It can soothe muscle tension and headaches and can help relieve insomnia. Massage is particularly beneficial after exercise. During a workout, waste products build up in the muscles. It can take the lymphatic system days to wash them away. Massage speeds up this process by improving the circulation of blood and lymph.

There are two main types of massage: shiatsu and Swedish. Shiatsu was developed in Japan at about the same time that acupuncture began to flourish in China. This massage involves finger pressure that stimulates the acupuncture points along the body's meridians. One form of shiatsu firmly massages certain areas of the body to stimulate the flow of energy and restore balance. Another form involves the use of a single fingertip to stimulate acupuncture points. The purpose of shiatsu is to alter the flow of energy within the body, and it works along the same principle as acupuncture. Shiatsu therapists also emphasize the importance of good nutrition and positive mental outlook, and they encourage clients to make lifestyle changes that promote greater health. Shiatsu can be combined with chiropractic to maximize its healing effects.

Swedish massage, which is more common in the West, involves four essential techniques, with the underlying premise that the hands should not lose contact with the body. Swedish massage is effective because of its continual, rhythmic motions. These are the basic techniques.

Effleurage: Rhythmic stroking with open hands, with movements directed toward the heart; this motion soothes and relaxes the body.

Percussion: Brisk rhythmic movements with alternate hands that include cupping, hacking (with sides of hands), pummeling (with fists), clapping, and plucking; this stimulates the skin and circulation.

Petrissage: Deep movement that involves lifting, rolling, squeezing, and pressing the skin; this stimulates muscles and fatty tissues, stretching taut muscles to relax them.

Pressure: As the thumbs, fingertips, or heel of the hand make small, pressured circular movements, friction stimulates superficial tissue.

When you visit a massage therapist, he or she probably will not take a detailed physical history, but you should inform him or her of any pains, illnesses, injuries, or recent surgeries you have had. The therapist usually will begin with the feet or back and will allow you a few moments to get used to the sensation of being touched and kneaded. It should be a thoroughly pleasurable treat!

Sessions are usually one hour long and cost approximately $30 to $70. Therapeutic massage is covered by some insurance companies when it is required by a doctor for the treatment of a particular ailment or injury due to an automobile or work-related accident. Massage is generally entirely safe, but you should not use it if the following conditions exist:

- Infectious, open wounds or bruises
- Varicose veins
- Fever
- Inflamed joints or acute arthritis
- Thrombosis or phlebitis (could disturb blood clot)

Reflexology

Reflexology is a technique of deeply massaging the soles of the feet and hands in order to affect various parts of the body that are ailing. It was developed in China and India at the same time that acupuncture originated. Reflexology was brought to England in the twentieth century by Dr. William Fitzgerald, who called it zone therapy. In the United States Eunice Ingham developed Fitzgerald's teachings in the 1930s. Today, reflexology is growing in popularity, with schools located in Europe and the United States. Many practitioners of reflexology also utilize chiropractic, osteopathy, and homeopathy.

Reflexology works on the premise that internal organs share the same nerve supplies as certain corresponding areas of the skin. Practitioners believe that the entire body is represented on the feet, primarily on the soles. By pressing the proper points on the feet, one can stimulate the organ associated with that point. These points are not the same as acupuncture points or meridians, many of which are not even represented on the feet.

During a reflexology session, the client will lie on a massage table while the practitioner feels the feet for granulelike substances deep within them. These "crystals" are actually waste deposits that build up in the nerve endings and capillaries and restrict the free flow of blood. The reflexology treatment breaks up the deposits so that they can be flushed from the body.

As the reflexologist "reads" the feet, he or she can determine which organs are affected. The patient will usually feel pain when a particular point is pressed, and sometimes in the corresponding organ or area of the body. The practitioner applies pressure with the edge of the thumb or finger and rotates it clockwise. The pressure is deep but should not be too painful. A session usually lasts from thirty to ninety minutes, and a client may require several sessions. Reflexology is beneficial for functional disorders that can be reversed, such as sinus problems, constipation, asthma, bladder problems, headaches, and stress.

PSYCHOTHERAPY

Psychotherapy, or "talk treatment," is an invaluable natural therapy for fostering and maintaining overall health. There has been much discussion about the mind/body connection. Although this has been an inherent part of holistic medicine throughout the world over time, orthodox Western medicine is realizing more and more the power of the mind and the importance of psychological treatments.

Mental health is important to physical health and vice versa. Emotional problems cause stress, which evokes physical symptoms and illness; physical illness, likewise, can cause a person to become depressed or lose energy and motivation. Doctors and patients are increasingly aware of the interplay of the mind and body and that in fact they may be inseparable, or one and the same.

Psychotherapy often requires you to talk about your feelings and problems, but it also can involve action, such as finding ways to alter your patterns of behavior. Treatment can be conducted on an individual basis between therapist and client, or it can be held within a group format. Group therapy allows clients to support and help each other, which can be just as valuable as receiving guidance from a therapist. People who seek out psychological treatment are not necessarily sick. They may simply be seeking greater understanding about themselves and their behavior.

There are many different kinds of psychotherapy, and some are more beneficial than others for treating particular disorders or problems. You may not hit upon the right therapy immediately, but don't give up. Success and progress in psychotherapy often take much time. If you really feel it's not working for you (and you've discussed this with the therapist), try a different therapist, and you might get better results. Psychotherapy, like many holistic, natural treatments, requires a willingness on the part of patients to be open to the treatment and to help themselves. You might go to a psychotherapist or counselor with the hope that the doctor will "cure" you. In fact, it takes work by both the therapist and the client in order for the treatment to be effective. The following sections list the major types of psychotherapy.

Supportive Psychotherapy

In this treatment, you can openly discuss your problems and feelings in a trusting, comfortable environment. The therapist should be a good listener who allows you the opportunity to vent your feelings, and who may make suggestions or point out insights that will give you a sense of support, without the feeling of being judged.

Exploratory Psychotherapy

This kind of treatment encourages you to explore your problems and issues, rather than just airing them. The therapist is usually active in the discussion and will let you know if you are avoiding a particular issue. Many healthy people pursue exploratory therapy as a way of learning more about themselves or to deal with a particular issue or aspect of their lives that they feel needs resolving or improvement.

Psychoanalysis

This treatment, which was originated by Sigmund Freud at the turn of the century, has taken a variety of forms. In classical psychoanalysis, you lie on a couch and talk freely about feelings, dreams, or whatever comes to mind. The psychoanalyst interprets what you say in terms of your childhood experiences and relationship with your parents. Psychoanalysis is usually intensive and long-term.

Other forms of psychoanalytic treatment focus on how your early emotional experiences have affected your current feelings and perceptions of yourself and relationships. This kind of therapy can help free you from pent-up or repressed childhood anger, frustration, hurt, and dependency. By working through these feelings, you will gain a greater sense of self-understanding and self-esteem.

Gestalt Therapy

Introduced in the United States by Fritz Perls in the 1950s, this "humanistic" therapy believes that the present moment, not the past, is most important, and that every person is responsible for his or her actions and has the ability to change them. In a session, if something from the past is bothersome, the therapist will help you bring it into the present. Gestalt therapists use many techniques to increase your awareness of yourself in the moment. For instance, if you are crying in a session, the therapist might ask you to speak to your tears. Merely talking about them promotes greater distancing between yourself and your emotions. Another Gestalt technique is for you to behave in a session opposite from the way you feel. For example, if you are very shy, the therapist might ask you to act like an outgoing person. Doing this will allow you to become aware of a part of yourself that exists but has remained undeveloped or repressed.

Behavioral Therapy

Behavioral therapists believe that all behavior is learned either through conditioning or the reinforcement of specific actions. For instance, if your mother taught you when you were growing up that all animals are dirty, you might develop a fear of animals, such as dogs. When the behavior you learned is negative or maladaptive, adverse psychological symptoms (in this example, a phobia) can result. Behavioral therapy can teach you new ways of behaving to help you live a more positive, happy, and productive life.

Behavioral therapy can resolve phobias, sexual dysfunction, inhibitions, and increase self-assertiveness. The therapist will help you learn new behaviors to replace those that are maladaptive. One method is called *operant conditioning,* by which new behaviors are rewarded and undesirable ones are ignored. In the *modeling* technique, the therapist "models," or displays for you to copy, the new behavior you are to practice. *Systemic desensitization* is a step-by-step process to help relieve specific fears or inhibitions.

Cognitive Therapy

This therapy was developed by American psychologist Aaron Beck in the 1960s. *Cognition* refers to a person's thinking, perception, and memory. If the therapist views your cognition as the cause of your emotional problems, the therapy will try to alter your perceptions and thoughts about yourself in order to alleviate the symptoms or problems. For example, if you were constantly denigrated by your father when you were growing up, chances are you developed a low self-esteem and often feel worthless. A cognitive therapist would point out evidence to the contrary, emphasizing your achievements that prove your self-worth.

Couples Therapy

Those who are married or involved in a serious intimate relationship know that even the best relationships require work. In couples therapy, you can visit a therapist either together or separately in order to understand and resolve tensions that exist within your relationship. Therapy can be useful to both heterosexual and homosexual couples.

Family Therapy

Families are intricate, dynamic networks that often require an objective outsider to help clear the air or resolve conflicts. When one or more family members has a problem, it often throws the entire unit into crisis, and this is when therapy can be beneficial. A family therapist is able to observe how the family operates together and can help the members understand not only how to deal with each other but their own roles within the family.

Just as it is important to find the right kind of therapy, it is equally important to build a good relationship with your therapist. As with other kinds of relationships, this can happen spontaneously, or it may take time. Within the emotional context of therapy, it is often difficult to discern how you feel about your therapist. Bear in mind that it is valid and important to discuss the feelings you have toward your therapist with him or her. This might reveal insight as to how you relate to others.

The different kinds of therapists are distinguished by their training. *Psychotherapist* is a general term that refers to anyone who practices psychotherapy. A *psychia-*

trist is a medical doctor who is trained in psychotherapy and can prescribe drugs for treating mental disorders. A *clinical psychologist* holds a doctoral degree in psychology and has training in psychotherapy. He or she cannot prescribe medicine, and may specialize in a particular type of therapy, such as psychoanalytic, behavioral, and so on. A *psychoanalyst* is a psychiatrist or psychologist who is specially trained in psychoanalysis.

You can seek psychotherapy from a private therapist or from a mental health center or clinic. Fees vary according to the practitioner, though some are willing to use a sliding scale—that is, they will charge a fee based on your income and the amount you are able to afford. Some insurance policies provide a psychotherapy benefit, while others do not. If your policy does, find out whether there is a limit to the number of sessions or if there is a cap on the amount of coverage provided each year.

BIOFEEDBACK

Biofeedback probably presents the greatest evidence of the mind's influence over the body. In a healthy person, physiological functions are performed and regulated by the brain and central nervous system. The mind, however, often interferes, such as under conditions of stress that produce tension in the body. Biofeedback can teach the patient to intervene under these conditions in order to restore balanced functioning in the body.

Conscious control can affect many body functions that can be measured accurately and continuously, such as heart rate, skin temperature, blood pressure, muscle tension, and brain waves. The biofeedback equipment that measures these functions includes the electroencephalograph (EEG), which records nerve and brain waves, the electromyograph (EMG), which registers muscle tension, and the galvanic skin resistance instrument (GSR), which detects the electrical conductivity of the skin to record states of arousal, excitement, or nervousness.

When you are hooked up to these machines, they convey information to you through signals that can be recognized and interpreted easily. For instance, when the instrument detects muscle tension, a red light might go on or a certain sound might be emitted to signal what is happening to you internally. You then can use this information, in addition to certain relaxation and imagery techniques, to begin controlling the muscle tension. The techniques that are used in combination with the biofeedback equipment include relaxation and autosuggestion exercises, visual imagery, and meditation. For example, if the equipment signals that your heart rate is increasing, you can use imagery, by imagining a calm, peaceful place, or meditate through the repeating of a mantra in order to relax your mind and body. In biofeedback treatment, therefore, the patient is not the object of the therapy, he or she *becomes* the therapy itself.

There are many applications for biofeedback, including stress-related illness, neuromuscular problems, and personal growth and increased self-awareness. Biofeedback can be effective treatment for emotional or behavioral problems, such as anxiety, depression, phobias, insomnia, tension headaches, and bruxism (teeth-grinding). It also can be used to treat illnesses considered by some professionals to be psychosomatic such as asthma, ulcers, colitis, diarrhea, cardiac arrhythmia, hypertension, Raynaud's syndrome, and migraines. Biofeedback can help victims of stroke, cerebral palsy, and muscle spasms in some functions of the muscles and movement. Since biofeedback increases your recognition and understanding of your total mind-body functioning, it also can be beneficial in enhancing personal growth and self-awareness.

Many general and psychiatric hospitals have biofeedback clinics, and it is probably best to undergo treatments administered by a psychologist who is trained in biofeedback. A psychologist would be helpful in the process of developing greater self-awareness, and you might even consider combining biofeedback with psychotherapy.

When you begin biofeedback sessions, you should be informed about the equipment being used and the learning process and receive information about the muscles and the physiological functions involved in the treatment. Having this knowledge will help you to relax during the treatment and will probably enhance its success. Remember that while you must be an active participant in biofeedback, too much effort can produce unwanted stress. The key is to relax using meditation, imagery, and other techniques, in order to focus fully on your internal states.

Biofeedback training can last weeks, months, or years, depending on your problem. Most people need at least six weeks' worth of sessions, which last from thirty to sixty minutes and can occur once a week or daily, again, depending on the need. The cost of biofeedback varies depending on your location, with an average cost of $75.00 per session. Check your insurance plan for coverage. You must learn to transfer what you learn from the biofeedback sessions to your daily life. It will take practice to begin to recognize the signs of trouble—such as muscle tension, headaches, and so on—and the situations in which they occur, and then to use the techniques that can relieve them without the biofeedback instrument. You probably will need periodic checkups in order to maintain the progress you have made.

NUTRITION

The value of good nutrition may be obvious, but it is often the obvious that is overlooked. If you do not eat the right foods, the organs and cells of your body will not get the nutrients they need to function and grow properly. Since food is a basic necessity, it also has been looked upon as essential medicine from very early times. People in ancient Greece and Egypt, for example, used garlic as a cure for respiratory infections, intestinal viruses, and skin conditions. Cabbage was a remedy for ulcers and headaches. In the 1700s, English ships began to carry lemons and limes to treat scurvy, a condition that affected sailors. It wasn't until the 1900s that scientists discovered the actual substance in citrus fruit that prevented scurvy. By this time, vitamin C had been isolated from lemons, and the first fat-soluble vitamin, A, was discovered.

By the 1940s, forty nutrients and thirteen vitamins had been isolated from foods. With the 1950s and 1960s came the era of processed foods, including the booming fast-food industry. This was followed in the next two decades by numerous fad diets as people desperately tried various ways to get rid of the weight gain that comes with this convenience.

Today, it seems that the public has a greater awareness of the kinds of things they ingest. New information on the dangers of substances such as pesticides, food additives, and saturated fats—and the benefits of nutrients—have altered the way many people eat. As you revamp your diet, however, it is important to read as much as you can in order to make informed choices about what you eat. Sometimes it is difficult to discern what is the latest fad and what is sound advice. Dieticians and nutritionists can help tailor your diet to your needs if you wish to pursue nutritional therapy to treat illness or allergies, or to bolster your health.

Essential Nutrients

All food is composed of certain substances that are necessary to maintain health: fats, proteins, carbohydrates, vitamins, minerals, and trace elements. Foods are characterized by categories (fat, carbohydrate, protein, dietary fiber), and a healthy diet balances a combination of them.

Protein

Approximately 17 percent of your body is composed of protein, including muscle, hair, bone, nails, and skin. Protein is also necessary for the production of hormones and enzymes. Since protein cannot be stored in the body, it must be absorbed regularly from foods such as milk, yogurt, cheese, eggs, meat, fish, sprouts, nuts, seeds, and legumes. If you do not eat enough protein, your muscles and tissues will degenerate. Too much protein, however, could strain the liver and kidneys and disrupts the balance

of minerals in your body. Protein should account for approximately 5 percent of your total caloric intake each
day.

Fats

Fat is an important source of energy. It helps to maintain organs, cell structure, nerves, and body temperature.
Fat also carries fat-soluble vitamins, such as A, D, E, and
K, around the body. There are three types of fatty acid:
saturated fat primarily comes from animal sources, such
as meat, fish, butter, cheese, eggs, and cream; *polyunsatu-
rated fat* comes from plant sources, such as wheat germ
and safflower, corn, and sunflower oils; *monounsaturated
fat* is found in olive oil, avocados, and peanuts. Saturated
fats, which can increase cholesterol levels, are the worst
kind of fat to consume. Most people in our society would
probably benefit from reducing their overall fat intake.
Fat should constitute no more than 30 percent of your
total daily caloric intake, with only 10 percent of this com-
ing from saturated fats.

Carbohydrates

Our main source of energy is carbohydrates, which are
converted into the glucose and glycogen that fuel muscles,
the brain, and the nervous system. Carbohydrates come
from starches and sugars. The best are starches in grains,
legumes, and pastas, and sugars in fruits and vegetables.
Refined sugar and flour contain high-calorie carbohydrates with little nutritional value. Unlike natural starches
and sugars, which convert into glucose more slowly and

are absorbed at a steady pace over time, they are absorbed quickly for instant bursts of energy. Carbohydrates should constitute the balance of your daily caloric intake (about 60 percent).

Dietary Fiber

Fiber, also referred to as roughage, is an indigestible substance found naturally in cereals, beans, nuts, vegetables, and fruits. Containing no nutrients and remaining undigested, it moves through the intestinal tract. As it absorbs liquid, it helps produce large soft stools that are easily passed. Fiber helps speed the passage of waste through the bowel and helps to remove toxic substances from the body. Low-fiber foods can take three or four days to pass through the digestive tract; high-fiber foods, in contrast, are usually passed within twenty-four hours. By consuming an adequate amount of fiber—and thus helping to move waste through the bowel more quickly— you may reduce your chances of developing colon cancer, diverticular disease, and gallstones.

Fiber occurs naturally in a wide variety of foods. Whole-grain cereals; whole-wheat, or bulgar-wheat, products; brown rice; barley; and bran are excellent sources of roughage. Legumes, oats, barley, and rye are also good sources and they form substances that restrict the amount of fat and sugar the body absorbs. This can help lower blood cholesterol levels and blood pressure. Corn, apples, carrots, brussels sprouts, eggplant, celery, potatoes, peas, and dried fruit are all good sources of dietary fiber. You should consume approximately one and one-half to two ounces (forty to sixty grams) of fiber each day.

Vitamins/Minerals

Vitamins and minerals are essential in aiding metabolism and the chemical processes in the body that release energy from food. The thirteen major vitamins are A, C, D, E, K, and eight B vitamins, often referred to as the B complex. Vitamins are soluble in either water or fat. Vitamin C and most of the B vitamins are water soluble. They must be consumed each day since they cannot be stored in the body. Any excess C or B vitamins are excreted. Vitamins A, D, E, and K are fat soluble, and they can be stored in the body's fatty tissues. Vitamin B_{12} can be stored in the liver.

Vitamins and minerals often work together and interact with each other. For example, vitamin C enhances the absorption of iron in the body. It is best to eat the daily required amounts of each vitamin and mineral in food.

If you decide to consult a nutritionist or dietician, he or she will help you devise a balanced diet and will recommend the supplements you should take according to any deficiencies you might have. If you are creating your own nutritional plan—or just modifying your eating habits—you should take a multivitamin and mineral supplement every day. This will ensure that you are getting the adequate amounts of nutrients that your body needs.

A Healthy Diet

Whole foods, or those produced with a minimal amount of processing, contain many of their original nutrients. Try to eat organically grown fruits and vegetables that have not been subject to chemical pesticides, meat and poultry that has not been given growth-hormone injections, and eggs from free-range chickens.

Generally, most people in our society need to eat more fruits and vegetables and to consume more fiber. It is best to eat fruits and vegetables raw and with their skins to ensure that you are getting all of their vitamins and minerals. Make sure to clean the skin thoroughly by scrubbing it with a brush (either a vegetable or pot-scrubbing brush) under running water to wash away unabsorbed chemicals from pesticides or other impurities. Fruits and vegetables should be eaten fresh, as they lose nutrients with age. They also lose nutrients through cooking, so try to cook them for as short a time and with as little liquid as possible. For example, if you usually boil vegetables, try steaming them instead. You'll probably enjoy their crispy texture and find that they have more taste! If you do boil your vegetables, consider using the liquid in stocks or sauces so as not to waste the vital nutrients.

Most of us also need to eat more fiber. If you now use white bread, try switching to whole-grain breads and cereals. Increase your fiber intake gradually in order to avoid a bloated feeling, which may occur temporarily.

If you want to consume less fat, eat only lean red meat in modest portions, and cook more poultry and fish. There are many good-quality low-fat products on the market, such as low-fat margarine. But use common sense in planning your diet. Remember that it is better to use just a little butter, a natural product, than to eat a lot of margarine, which contains added chemicals and hydrogenated fats. You also should consider using skim milk and low-fat yogurt and cheese. Avoid eating rich desserts, such as ice cream or pastries, fried foods, and rich sauces.

Most of us can probably do with less sugar and salt in our diets. Refined white sugar has no nutritional value, so try cutting down your use of it. If your sweet tooth will not be denied, replace sugar with honey or fruit juices— they are natural sweeteners. Try eating fruit or sugarless baked goods and jams that are sweetened only with fruit juices.

Although some salt is necessary, most people consume too much of it since it is used in excess in many processed foods. Remember, salt occurs naturally in many foods, so there is no reason to add more. Substitute herbs and spices for salt when you are cooking, and try to eat fewer processed foods. Generally, you should consume one ounce (twenty-five grams) or less of sugar and less than one-fourth ounce (six grams) of salt each day.

It was discovered long ago that honey and salt could help preserve foods. Over the past few decades, the use of artificial additives and preservatives has increased greatly, replacing the natural ones. Some of these are harmless in small amounts, and some additives even occur naturally, such as monosodium glutamate (MSG) in fermented soy products (soy sauce). However, when restaurants add excess amounts of MSG in the preparation of food, some people experience adverse physical symptoms, such as headaches, nausea, and dizziness.

Dyes, preservatives, stabilizers, antioxidants, and emulsifiers are all food additives that can cause reactions in people who are sensitive to these substances. Most additives are thoroughly tested for safety, and they must be listed on each product, according to the rules of the Food and Drug Administration (FDA). They are not all bad, but some people are particularly sensitive to them, and they can adversely affect hyperactive children.

In order to test your own sensitivity, or that of your child, to certain additives, you need to begin a very restricted diet of bland basic foods. Gradually reintroduce one at a time those foods that are suspect and record any reactions. It is best to consult a nutritionist, naturopath, or doctor who specializes in food sensitivities when conducting a test such as this.

The best advice for planning good nutrition is to avoid foods that you know you are allergic to and to maintain a balanced diet. Eat low-fat, high-fiber, naturally sweetened foods, and let moderation and common sense be your guide.

Calorie Chart

The word *calorie* refers to a unit of energy. Calories represent the amount of energy needed to burn a particular substance. The number of calories each person needs for maximum energy depends on age, sex, occupation, and lifestyle. The following chart serves as a guide for the amount of daily caloric intake for various groups of people:

MEN

Age	*Lifestyle*	*Calories Needed Daily*
18–35	Inactive	2,500
	Active	3,000
	Very active	3,500

Age	Lifestyle	Calories Needed Daily
36–70	Inactive	2,400
	Active	2,800
	Very active	3,400

WOMEN

Age	Lifestyle	Calories Needed Daily
18–55	Inactive	1,900
	Active	2,100
	Very active	2,500
56–70	Inactive	1,700
	Active	2,000

In their quest for health, fitness, and the perfect body, many people become almost obsessive about counting calories. Remember that it is not so much the number of calories you consume, but where they come from, that is important. In other words, it is better to eat 400 calories' worth of pasta and vegetables than of ice cream. The key to planning and following a healthy diet is balance. Eat a variety of whole foods from the basic food groups, and eliminate or moderate your consumption of those foods that you know are not good for you.

Orthomolecular Medicine

Ortho is the Greek word meaning "to correct." Two-time Nobel prize winner Linus Pauling coined the term *orthomolecular medicine* in 1968 to refer to a system of correcting the body's metabolism with the right combination of nutrients, such as vitamins, minerals, amino acids, and enzymes. All of these nutrients occur naturally in the body as a defense against illness, but sometimes the body becomes deficient in one or many of them.

In 1943, the National Resource Council's Food and Nutrition Board established the Recommended Dietary Allowances (RDAs) of various nutrients. In 1963, the Food and Drug Administration created minimum daily requirements called U.S. RDAs, which are used by food manufacturers. The levels of U.S. RDAs are based on the lowest levels necessary to prevent known diseases, such as scurvy, which are caused by deficiencies. However, these levels are not necessarily high enough to promote health and combat other common illnesses. Orthomolecular doctors and other scientists advocate setting nutritional standards not based on avoiding diseases such as scurvy, but on promoting optimum health.

Orthomolecular medicine is holistic in that it considers mental and physical causes of biochemical imbalances in the body. Practitioners perform blood tests and use vitamin and mineral profiles to delineate levels for sixteen vitamins and thirty minerals. Many physical and mental disorders can be treated simply by supplementing deficiencies in these nutrients.

Since each individual is unique, each has different nutritional needs. People who take megadoses of nutrients should take breaks from their dosages in order to prevent overdose. Orthomolecular treatments should be supervised by a trained doctor or nutritionist.

EXERCISE

Most of us live rather sedentary lives—we drive instead of walking or riding a bike; we sit at work; and we watch television while resting on the couch. Yet exercise is vital to our physical and emotional health. It improves muscle tone and posture, increases strength and stamina, and can improve circulation and respiration. Not only does exercise reduce blood-fat levels, it can change large blood-fat globules (low-density lipoproteins) to smaller, less sticky ones (high-density lipoproteins) that move more easily and are less likely to clog arteries. Exercise also is good for the mind. It invigorates and energizes, and helps to relieve tension and anxiety. By helping to release substances that affect emotions, such as adrenaline and noradrenaline, exercise can even relieve the symptoms of depression. Have you ever heard of a runner's high? The explanation for runners' "addiction" to their exercise is that it helps to release endorphins and enkephalins, which have a mood-elevating effect. When you exercise, your body gets in shape and your mind begins to relax.

There are several different kinds of exercise, and a good workout routine should include a little of each. *Isotonic* exercises, such as weight training, stretching, and yoga, develop muscle strength and flexibility. They do not have the aerobic benefits of improving respiration and circulation, but they are essential for toning slack muscles and building strength. *Stretching* exercises, as part of your warmup and cool-down, are a must in any kind of workout.

Aerobics refer to sustained exercise that increases the amount of oxygenated blood carried to muscles and organs. In other words, any activity that increases your breathing and heart rate is aerobic: aerobic dance, step aerobics, running, jogging, fitness walking, cycling, swimming, and cross-country skiing. Stationary bicycles, Lifecycles, and StairMasters are aerobic fitness machines. When you perform an aerobic exercise, you should maintain your training-level heart rate for fifteen minutes or longer in order to receive maximum results. (See the chart on pages 70–1.) Aerobic exercise improves the respiratory and circulatory systems. It strengthens the heart muscle, makes arteries and veins more elastic, and lowers blood-fat and body-fat levels.

Anaerobic exercise is the opposite of aerobic exercise. It is characterized by short bursts of energy, such as sprinting. Although anaerobic exercise does develop muscle strength, it does not improve circulation and respiration.

When you plan an exercise regimen, consider activities that you enjoy, that are feasible, and that you will want to do. That way you'll have a better chance of maintaining your exercise routine. Some people like to exercise alone —it is "quiet" time to think or clear the mind. Others prefer to exercise with a partner or a group because other people can be a good source of motivation and can make exercise a fun social event. You also need to consider how much time you can allot to the activity. When you have a very busy schedule, it is easy to forgo the exercising, especially if you are tired. Just try to remember that the more you exercise, the more energy you will have in the long run for all of your life's activities.

If you are over the age of forty and have been relatively inactive, are pregnant, or have another medical condition, you should consult a physician and have a complete physical exam before beginning an exercise program. When you start, begin slowly and gradually increase the duration and intensity of your workouts. Warming up is a must—stretch your muscles slowly and smoothly for at least five minutes. The endurance phase of your workout should last approximately twenty to thirty minutes, getting your pulse rate up to training level. Cooling down is also imperative—spend five to ten minutes walking briskly and doing more stretching exercises.

The following chart will help you determine your training-level pulse rate. The resting pulse of adults is generally sixty to eighty beats per minute. To take your pulse, use the first three fingers of your hand to feel the beat in your temple or neck. Count the number of beats in fifteen seconds and multiply that by four to equal one minute.

Age	Beats per minute for Training Level
20	138–158
25	137–156
30	135–154
35	134–153
40	132–151
45	131–150
50	129–147
55	127–146
60	126–144
65	125–142
70	123–141
75	122–139

Age	Beats per minute for Training Level
80	120–138
85	119–136

Once you get into the swing of an exercise routine, you'll probably look forward to the activities—and even feel bad if you skip a session. Remember to use common sense when you are exercising, especially if you do strenuous aerobic activity. Here are some tips:

- Do not exercise if you are ill, dizzy, or feel faint. If any of these feelings occur during a workout, cool down by walking and stretching, and then take off a day or two.

- Do not exercise if you feel severe muscle or joint pain; take a few days off and begin again gradually. If pain persists, consult a physician.

- Always warm up and cool down to avoid stiff or injured muscles.

- Allow two hours after meals before exercising.

- Avoid exercising in very hot weather and dress warmly in cold weather if you exercise outside; even if you perspire, keep all of your clothing on to avoid chilled muscles that can result in cramps or pulls.

- "No pain, no gain" may be true to a degree, but you should build the intensity of your workout gradually. Use common sense, listen to your body and mind, and don't overdo it!

CHAPTER THREE

Mental Health and the Mind/Body Connection

What is mental health? What does it mean to be mentally ill? How does one develop a mental disorder, or go from health to illness? Psychology, or the study of the mind, is a fascinating but inexact science. Although it is difficult with many mental illnesses to determine the exact cause, most psychologists and natural medicine practitioners agree that there are physiological, social, genetic, and environmental factors involved in the development of mental disorders. Since the 1950s, enormous progress has been made in understanding these various factors as well as in the development of drugs to help control the biochemical imbalances. In some cases, medications are necessary to correct the biological aspects of mental disorders. Other cases simply require a reduction of stressors that may be causing the problem. Whether it is used solely or to complement traditional drug treatment, natural medicine can sometimes restore your biological and psychological balance in order to alleviate your condition.

Although allopathic medicine is increasingly acknowledging the connection between the mind and body, natural medicine has always recognized the importance of the mind and the role that it plays in health. In fact, it is the mind—the deepest level of existence—that is most important to treat when you are trying to achieve a cure from any kind of illness, either physical or mental.

The mind is crucial on both the physiological and psychological levels. It is embodied and empowered by the brain, nerves, and hormones, which if thrown off balance send the mind into a state of disarray. Psychological or psychosocial factors such as early learning, conditioning, and stress can sometimes trigger biological imbalances. Natural medicine, being holistic, treats both the physiological and psychological aspects of mental illness, either alone or in combination with traditional drug therapy. Healthy people also can use many alternative treatments to prevent mental disorders from developing.

HISTORICAL VIEWS OF
MENTAL ILLNESS

The oldest records about behavior can be found in the writing of Plato, the Bible, and the Babylonian king Hammurabi (1750 B.C.), which all point to evil spirits as the cause of abnormality. This belief prevailed from Hammurabi's time to the 1700s, and treatment to drive out evil spirits included chanting, prayer, and the use of purgatives to induce vomiting. In the Middle Ages (A.D. 500 to 1500) the Catholic Church published *Witches' Hammer* (*Malleus Maleficarum* in Latin), which detailed descriptions of exorcisms. These procedures, aimed at driving out the "devil" from a "possessed" person, began with prayers and eventually included torture if the treatment was failing. If torture proved unsuccessful, the person was set afire in order to save his or her soul from the devil.

Hippocrates was one of the first physicians to claim that biological imbalances—not demons—produced mental illness. Believing that the body was composed of four fluids, or "humors"—blood, phlegm, black bile, and yellow bile—he thought that imbalances among these fluids were at fault. Although this theory was proven untrue, it was a precursor for later theories regarding other natural causes for mental disorders.

In the 1800s, the German physician Richard von Krafft-Ebing discovered that a severe psychological disturbance known as "paresis" was actually a late stage of syphilis. Therefore, in the case of paresis at least, a biological cause for a mental disorder was finally firmly established. Up to this point, physicians tended to steer clear of mental illness, but with this newfound evidence for biological causality, they became more involved in the treatment and care of mentally ill people. Doctors began to be installed as heads of mental institutions, and the practice of psychiatry was formed. However, although a biological cause was found for paresis, causes for other mental disorders have been more elusive. While there is evidence of physiological differences between mentally healthy and mentally ill individuals, it is difficult to pinpoint exact physical causes for mental disorders, and most contemporary scientists believe that psychological factors are involved as well.

Pythagoras, the ancient Greek father of geometry, believed in psychological causes of mental illness. He would send his patients to "temples" where they could rest, exercise, and eat right. He also recognized the value of talk therapy and provided people with the opportunity to speak to understanding people who would listen to their problems and give advice on how to improve their lives. Throughout time there have been other proponents of the psychological factors involved in abnormal behavior, but these ideas did not really gain recognition until Sigmund Freud formulated his theories of personality development and conscious and unconscious behavior.

Like Pythagoras, natural medicine practitioners recognize the importance of psychosocial and environmental factors in the development of mental illnesses. Stress, anxiety, irrational fears, sleep disturbances, and depression are all disorders that you can control or prevent by proper care of your mind. Psychotherapy, biofeedback, relaxation techniques, herbal medicine, and other alternative treatments can help you overcome mental problems and cope with the factors that contribute to them.

HOW DOES THE MIND BECOME ILL?

Mental health is characterized by the ability to cope with a wide range of situations and events that run the gamut from happy and pleasant to sad and tragic. If, during your life, you have developed ways to handle stress effectively—or if you are able to locate and eliminate its cause when it arises—you are probably a mentally healthy person. If, however, you have not learned ways to handle life's stresses effectively, you could develop thoughts, feelings, or behavior that prevent you from living a productive, content life.

Your mind thus can become ill as a result of certain social and environmental conditions. How you were raised, your relationships with your parents and siblings, and the way you learned to think and behave can affect how you relate to and function in the world as an adult. For instance, if your parents were extremely demanding and critical of you when you were growing up, you might be a perfectionist or overachiever. As an adult, you are very hard on yourself, pressuring yourself to perform, achieve, and be the best in all you do. If you allow this self-inflicted stress to continue unchecked, it could lead to an anxiety disorder or depression.

Likewise, consider your parents' attitudes when you were growing up. Were they worriers? Were they the kind of people who always saw the glass as being half empty? If so, you may tend to think negatively too, since this attitude has been instilled in you. Did your parents constantly fight when you were young? If so, you've probably learned that this is the way to deal with conflicts and problems. Similarly, research shows that if you were raised in an abusive environment—involving physical, verbal, or emotional abuse—you are more likely be an abuser. The kind of environment and atmosphere you are raised in, therefore, has a profound effect on your way of thinking and behaving.

Socialization is another crucial factor that contributes to mental health and adaptability. Have you always made friends easily, or are you a loner? Were your parents supportive of you as a child and teenager? Did you have close solid relationships with other family members? A social network is important in helping you both to cope with hardships or to celebrate triumphs. If you did not have strong social support as a child, you may tend to be more withdrawn as an adult too. You may feel that it is important, above all else, to be independent, and you may not be able to ask others for help. This kind of social isolation or distance can contribute to the development of emotional or mental problems.

Finally, the mind also can become ill due to physical illness or injury. For example, a brain injury, caused by a severe blow or trauma to the head, could trigger a mental condition such as emotional instability, loss of voluntary control over behavior, or memory lapses, depending on the area of the brain that is affected. Certain diseases can affect the brain, thereby causing mental imbalances. These illnesses include stroke, Parkinson's disease, AIDS-related dementia, Alzheimer's disease, and hyperthyroidism.

The precise *causes* of specific mental disorders are not known, but it is clear that a combination of social, environmental, and biological factors are involved in the development of mental illness. While you cannot change or erase the past experiences that have contributed to your own mental status, you certainly can learn to change your behavior, ways of thinking, and ways of handling stress in order to restore or maintain good mental health. When your mind becomes ill in any way—whether it is just "stressed out" or suffers from a more severe mental disorder—your entire being suffers. Holistic medicine, understanding the importance and vitality of the mind, offers a wide range of treatments for keeping it in good health.

THE MIND

In order to understand mental illnesses and how they can be treated, it is essential to discuss first the broader subject of the mind. What is the mind? How and when does it begin to function? Despite modern knowledge and technology, the mind remains somewhat mysterious to even the most astute philosophers and doctors. Chinese doctors see the mind as *chi;* homeopaths call it our vital force. We can begin to unravel the mystery of the mind by considering how it is embodied by the brain.

Generally speaking, we use the word "mind" to refer to things such as cognition, memory, feelings, intelligence, reason, perception, and judgment. We think of the brain as the counterpart upon which the mind depends in order to function. The brain, in turn, relies on the hormones, chemicals, and nerve cells as they exist and travel throughout the body. The mind, therefore, appears to inhabit the entire body, both in a physical and spiritual sense.

You can view the mind from a physiological standpoint, as it is embodied by the brain and nervous system, or from a metaphysical perspective, as an energy that pervades the body and makes us each unique individuals. However you wish to define the mind, it is clear that it plays a major role in both physical and mental illnesses, a role that natural medicine sees as supreme. The mind, or the deepest level of being, is the basis of health, and if it becomes ill, it can trigger both physical and psychological symptoms. To practitioners and followers of natural medicine, sound mental health is vital to overall well-being.

In order to fully understand the concept of mind as

well as the development of mental disorders, it is necessary to explore the physiological components of the mind. These are, of course, the brain and the rest of the nervous system as well as the endocrine system.

THE BRAIN

The brain is a complex mass of nerve cells, or neurons, that has the capacity to think, calculate, feel, regulate, and communicate. Although it is composed of specialized parts, it operates as a single unit with all parts working together.

The hindbrain is the lowest portion of the brain, located at the base of the skull. It is responsible for routine functions that keep the body in proper working order. The hindbrain is composed of the medulla, the swelling at the top of the spinal cord that controls breathing and reflexes, and the cerebellum, a mass behind the medulla that maintains muscle coordination and tone.

The midbrain, a small area at the top of the hindbrain, serves as a relay center for messages from the eyes and ears. The forebrain, which fills most of the skull, includes the thalamus, hypothalamus, and cerebral cortex. The thalamus routes messages from the body to the appropriate parts of the brain. The hypothalamus is involved in motives, emotions, and the involuntary function of internal organs. It is especially important in regulating body temperature, sleep, endocrine gland activity, secretions in the stomach and intestines, and the rhythm of the heartbeat. The cerebral cortex controls conscious experience and intelligence, and it is involved with the voluntary nervous system. It is divided into two halves, or hemispheres, joined by a structure that facilitates communications between them, called the corpus callosum.

THE NERVOUS SYSTEM

The brain is the major organ of the nervous system. It is connected to a thick bundle of nerves, called the spinal cord, that runs throughout the spine. Individual nerves branch out from the spinal cord to every part of the body, carrying messages from the body to the brain and vice versa. The brain and spinal cord compose the central nervous system, and the nerves branching off the spinal cord constitute the peripheral nervous system. These nerves are composed of cells called neurons that relay messages along the nerve in a fascinating way.

An individual neuron is composed of a cell body, with dendrites, rootlike structures, that branch off it. The dendrites receive messages from other neurons and pass them on to the cell body. Each neuron also has an axon, another structure that branches off the cell body, which carries messages away from the cell body and transmits them via electrical impulses to the next neuron. The dendrites and axons are covered by a layer called the myelin sheath, which insulates the neuron and helps conduct the electrical impulses. It speeds up the conduction by allowing the impulse to skip over gaps in the sheath rather than traveling the entire length of the neuron.

Neurons are not directly connected but are linked in chains. The space between two neurons is called a synapse, and the electrical impulses cross over the synapse.

Their ability to do this depends on neurotransmitters, chemicals released from the tips of dendrites across the synapse. The neurotransmitter stimulates the adjacent dendrite to help move the impulse along to the next neuron.

Different neurotransmitters work in different parts of the brain. Some are excitatory, allowing the neuron to transmit the electrical impulse, while others are inhibitory, preventing the conduction. Given the specificity of neurotransmitter action in the brain, medications have been successful in treating neurotransmitter imbalances, particularly in mental disorders such as depression and anxiety.

The general term "nervous system" really refers to two different systems. The voluntary nervous system controls conscious voluntary processes, such as movement and language. The autonomic, or involuntary, nervous system controls the actions of internal organs, such as heartbeat, breathing, digestion, sweating, and sexual arousal. It also regulates emotions, which is why there is often a physical component to an extreme emotional state, such as headache, a pounding heart, or stomachache. During a period of intense emotion, the autonomic nervous system overextends itself, throwing various organs off balance.

The autonomic nervous system is divided into two parts. The sympathetic nervous system activates the internal organs during emotional arousal; the parasympathetic nervous system calms the organs afterward. These two parts work together to maintain the overall balance and function of the body's organs.

The voluntary and autonomic nervous systems are somewhat linked in the brain so that thoughts can influence emotions and vice versa. Although the autonomic system is difficult to control consciously, you can learn to influence it yourself, as well as learn to regulate your emotions and relax your body. You can learn to regulate some of these functions through biofeedback, a natural treatment discussed in detail in Chapter 4.

THE ENDOCRINE SYSTEM

We've spoken about how the nervous system transmits messages throughout the body. But what exactly are these messages? What are they composed of? The answer lies in the chemicals known as hormones.

The endocrine system encompasses all of the glands that secrete hormones, chemical messengers that control internal organs. The adrenal glands secrete epinephrine, which increases the heart rate, and norepinephrine, which raises blood pressure, increases metabolism, causes the liver to release stored sugar into the bloodstream, and slows digestion. When you are under stress, the adrenal glands step up their production of these hormones to help your body deal with the stressor.

The islets of Langerhans, glands embedded in the pancreas, regulate blood sugar through two hormones. Glucagon causes the liver to convert stored sugar into blood sugar and dump it into the bloodstream. Insulin reduces blood sugar by helping the cells to absorb it from the blood more easily. Blood-sugar level is an important factor that determines how energetic a person feels.

The thyroid gland, located below the voice box, regulates metabolism. It secretes thyroxin, a hormone necessary for proper mental development to occur in children. In adults, it helps to determine activity and weight. Four small parathyroid glands within the thyroid secrete parathormone, which is necessary for the proper function of the nervous system.

The pituitary gland, found near the bottom of the brain, has perhaps the biggest job of all. It secretes hormones that regulate the activity of the other glands, as well as hormones that affect blood pressure, thirst, and growth.

DEVELOPMENT OF THE BRAIN AND MIND

As a human body grows in utero, the brain is present before birth and develops throughout the course of a lifetime. It is most full of nerve cells at birth; thereafter a continual attrition of these cells occurs. There is also a slow ongoing loss of connections between the nerve cells and neurotransmitters. Therefore, as one gets older, fewer messages are sent, fewer neurotransmitters exist to send the messages, and there are fewer receptor branches to receive them. While you can function with progressively fewer neurons, your functioning becomes less efficient. To compensate for the loss of nerve cells, healthy brain cells grow more dendrites, or nerve branches, to foster communication between nerve cells. Although there are fewer neurons, they become more active and make new connections. As a person grows and develops, he or she loses cells with age, and the brain adapts to make the most of what it has.

Despite these losses in the brain brought on by age, intellect remains intact. "Crystallized intelligence"—vocabulary, comprehension, and overall knowledge—does not decline much because of an aging brain. However, "fluid intelligence"—memory span and the ability to process information quickly—is affected by age. As you grow older, your reaction time increases, your recall of information is not as good, and your information processing is slower. Endurance, strength, and coordination are often diminished as well. Every individual experiences age differently, however. Although functions, capacities, and skills diminish, the mind, which is flexible and adaptable, can use the experience and wisdom it has amassed to compensate for these losses. In this sense, age really is just a state of mind.

Sometimes disease impairs the brain during the normal aging process. In such a case, you may become disoriented, clumsy, and suffer from rambling speech and an inability to recognize others. These symptoms are among those seen in dementia, which affects approximately three million people in the United States. Many instances of dementia stem from causes that can be reversed, such as depression, thyroid disease, vitamin deficiencies, and the side effects of medication. Strikingly, 55 to 60 percent of dementia victims suffer from Alzheimer's disease, a progressive, irreversible, degenerative illness named for the German psychiatrist Alois Alzheimer, who identified the disease at the turn of the century. Because of the disease, the impairment of neurons is grossly accelerated, and other changes in the brain cause it to shrink, thereby eroding many mental functions.

There are two categories of Alzheimer's disease. Senile

dementia of the Alzheimer's type (SDAT), which begins in a person's late sixties or early seventies, is the most common. Presenile dementia occurs in people in their fifties to early sixties and is characterized by a more rapid degeneration. The first symptoms of Alzheimer's disease are progressive memory loss, depression, mood swings, disorientation, personality changes, and physical problems. The illness is diagnosed based on symptoms and the elimination of other possibilities, since there are no definitive laboratory tests to diagnose it at this time.

The causes of Alzheimer's disease are as yet unknown. Genetic factors may be involved; some researchers believe that it is caused by a slow virus, one that enters the body long before symptoms occur. Since older people tend to have weaker immune systems, they are less able to defend against viruses. An interesting fact is that Alzheimer's patients have 60 to 90 percent less of the enzymes that synthesize acetylcholine, a neurotransmitter essential for memory. It is possible that other neurotransmitter systems also may be involved in the disease.

Although the process of aging does involve the loss of brain nerve cells and diminished functions and capacities, several factors influence how each individual copes with it. Environment and lifestyle are major factors in mental and physical health, particularly during old age. Remaining active in work and social activities provides a sense of purpose and self-reliance, and exercising the mind and body will help to maintain mental sharpness and clarity. Unfortunately, many elderly people find themselves alone, suffering illnesses, facing financial burdens, dealing with the loss of spouses or loved ones, and fearing death. This causes frequent cases of depression, which can be alleviated through social support networks such as groups and housing developments for senior citizens.

Finally, there is probably no greater complication to a healthy aging process than stress. Although everyone is exposed to it, stress affects only certain people adversely —those who have not found constructive, positive ways to cope with it. As mentioned earlier, when you are under stress, your adrenal glands secrete hormones called gluco-corticoids that help your body to deal with the tension. Too much glucocorticoids can make you sick, causing chronic high blood pressure and even killing brain cells. Chronic stress often results when you feel that you are not in control or are unable to predict events. It is important to learn to relax, to take things in stride, since times when you just can't be in control, when things don't go exactly as you planned, are inevitable.

Stress plays a major role not only in the aging process but in overall health and immunity. The effects of stress on your body and mind are discussed in greater detail in the following chapter.

Chapter Four

Stress and Your Health

All of us at one time or another have felt "stressed out." But when stress becomes a chronic condition of your life, it's time to do something about it. Chronic stress can and will cause psychological and physical illness if it continues to persist untreated.

It is clear that prolonged stress and the body's reaction to it gradually weaken vital organs and systems. Chronic elevated blood pressure can damage the heart, kidneys, and cardiovascular system; increased blood sugar raises cholesterol levels; buildup of plaque clogs arteries; increased acid in the stomach can cause ulcers and gastrointestinal problems; an overworked system will lead to chronic fatigue and insomnia. Chronic stress also has a very adverse effect on the immune system, which helps the body fight infections and disease.

In addition to these physical problems, stress can affect your mind in the form of anxiety or depression. Chronic stress and your mind can become engaged in a vicious cycle that feeds upon itself and causes mental health to decline. For example, imagine that you have just bought a new home and the mortgage payments are tough to make. On top of that, the house is in need of repairs. You're very stressed out about these new responsibilities, and the pressure is starting to get you down. You feel despondent and don't feel like socializing; you've taken a second job, but this just compounds the stress. You feel exhausted and pessimistic, and begin to blame yourself for doing something wrong—after all, other people manage to own new homes. What's wrong with you? This self-criticism will make you feel even worse about yourself and your situation. It's a cycle of stress, worry, and depression—which you can turn on yourself or take out on others—and it only serves to drag you in a downward spiral.

Stress's effect on your mind—the way you think and feel—is as damaging as its effect on your body. While it is easy to recover from isolated stressful events—such as a bad day at work or a fight with your spouse—persistent stress can almost seem to change your personality. You might become irritable or depressed or even hostile to others. You might even develop other anxiety-related disorders, such as agoraphobia, obsessive or compulsive behavior, or generalized anxiety disorder.

CAUSES OF STRESS

Natural medicine, from its holistic viewpoint, recognizes a host of stressors in people's lives. Undue pressure at home or work, financial burdens, exposure to extreme climates or hostile environments, loss of loved ones, physical or emotional abuse . . . if you think about your own life, you probably can add many more stressors to this list.

The sources of stress are not always obvious. Even joyous events, such as a wedding, a job promotion, buying a new home, or the birth of a child, can cause much stress.

You also might get stressed out if you cannot achieve a particular goal or satisfy a certain wish. For instance, you may want very much to have a child but cannot conceive. Fertility tests can't elucidate any reasons for this, and you feel very frustrated—why is this happening to you? Certainly this is a very emotional issue—and one that you do not have much control over—that can cause much stress in your life.

Stress also exists in tandem with the pressure you feel when you perceive that negative consequences are attached to your actions. For instance, you might feel pressured to maintain a certain level of performance at work or else risk getting fired. If you find yourself thinking in this way, you should stop and consider whether the threat is real or if you are just being too hard on yourself. You might be able to control and even eliminate this kind of stress from your life.

Stress also stems from conflict, which is not always negative. For instance, a conflict could occur in having to choose between two positive goals of equal value, such as choosing between two excellent job offers. Or your conflict could involve a choice that has both a positive and negative outcome, such as you're getting married but it necessitates your moving across the country away from family and friends.

Numerous life events—such as the death of a family member or friend, the loss of a job, buying a house or moving, having a child—cause stress. Two U.S. Navy physicians, Thomas Holmes and Richard Rahe, developed a list of major life stressors. These are listed in descending order, beginning with the most stressful event:

Death of a spouse
Divorce
Marital separation
Imprisonment
Death of a close relative
Personal injury or illness
Marriage
Fired from a job
Marital reconciliation
Retirement
Illness of a relative
Pregnancy
Sexual problems
Birth or adoption
Business readjustment
Change in financial status
Death of a close friend
Change to different work
Increased arguments with spouse
Mortgage or loan for major purchase
Foreclosure on mortgage or loan
Change in job responsibilities
Child leaving home
Problems with in-laws
Outstanding personal achievement
Spouse begins or stops work
Begin or end school
Change in living conditions
Changing personal habits
Problems with your boss
Change in work hours/conditions
Change in residence or school

Recreation
Church or social activities
Mortgage or loan for smaller purchase
Change in sleeping habits
Change in family gatherings
Change in eating habits
Vacation
Christmas
Minor law violations

Read through these items again and consider how many of them apply to yourself at the given moment, or within the past six months. You might be surprised by the number of stressors you are dealing with!

HOW STRESS BEGINS

Stress, especially when it becomes chronic, can suppress your immune system and lead to physical diseases, and it can contribute to the development of mental disorders. The circumstances during which the stress occurs and your attitude toward it are critical to how you will handle the stress. The time of day, frequency, duration, and cause of the stress are all conditions that contribute to your reaction to it.

Stress usually begins as a reaction to your environment or relationships. All individuals have expectations that are based on their upbringing, education, and so on, and each person perceives situations according to these expectations. If the events or relationships do not live up to the person's expectations, he or she will probably begin to question what is wrong. If he or she cannot justify or change the situation, stress begins to build.

In order to understand the pervasive nature of stress, consider the following situation. You have just been interviewed for a job that you really want. You thought the interview went well, but it has been one week and the company has not called you back. You begin to wonder what is taking so long—was it something you said or did in the interview? You start to go over and over the interview in your mind, trying to recall each detail. Your mind becomes preoccupied with trying to figure out what you perceive to be a problem. In reaction to this stress, your brain sends messages to your muscles to tighten up and get ready to react. The body responds with signals, such as headaches, backaches, stomachaches, anxiety, or insomnia, but your mind is so preoccupied with the problem that it is more or less oblivious to the adverse effects of the building tension. In this example, of course, the cause of the stress most likely will be resolved in a short time. But if the situation caused prolonged stress, it is clear just how damaging it could be to the mind and body.

YOUR BODY'S RESPONSE
TO STRESS:
FIGHT OR FLIGHT

When chronic stress remains untreated, it triggers biological changes in the body. These changes, known as the "general adaption syndrome," consist of three phases—alarm, resistance, and exhaustion—representing the body's mechanism for coping with stress. The general adaption syndrome is regulated by the adrenal glands, which are responsible for maintaining the balance of body functions.

Any disturbance of the normal hormone secretion of the adrenal glands affects your response to stress. For instance, if your adrenal glands are sluggish, you will probably feel "stressed out" and may be prone to developing allergies. If your adrenal activity is abnormally high, it could cause high blood pressure, anxiety, depression, and high blood sugar and cholesterol levels.

The general adaption syndrome illustrates the influence that your mind and body have on each other. When you experience stress, your adrenal glands and the general adaption mechanism kick into action. If this adrenal activity continues for a prolonged period of time because of persistent stress, it could cause chronic anxiety or even depression. You can see how the mind and body are inextricably linked, and why natural medicine, which gives equal weight to both aspects of the person, is so effective in treating and preventing illness.

The alarm stage of the general adaption syndrome is referred to as the fight-or-flight response. As your experience of stress begins to build, your brain and endocrine system are stimulated to secrete adrenaline and other stress-related hormones. These help prepare your body to take action, if necessary—either to fight the perceived stress or flee from it.

During the fight-or-flight response, several physiological changes occur. Your heart rate increases, pumping blood to all body parts in preparation for their reaction to stress. Your body begins to perspire in order to lower its temperature, digestive activities slow down, and the liver

dumps glucose into the blood. All of these changes help
your body mobilize energy in preparation for its reaction
to stress.

All of us have experienced the fight-or-flight response
at one time or another. Have you ever, for instance, had
to give a speech to a group of colleagues? Unless you're a
natural-born ham, you probably felt nervous or anxious
about it. You had butterflies in your stomach, your an-
tiperspirant just wasn't working, and when you reached
the podium, your heart began to race. These are all signals that your body was preparing to handle the stress
caused by the situation.

The fight-or-flight response is a short phase and is
often sufficient to cope with a given stressor. Afterward,
your body will rest in order to restore balance. However,
if the stress continues, your body enters the phase of resistance, which allows it to continue its struggle with the
stressor at hand. Corticosteroids are important in the resistance phase. For example, glucocorticoids help convert
protein to energy; mineralocorticoids promote sodium re-
tention, which keeps the blood pressure elevated. With
increased energy and circulation, the body can continue
to deal with stress. However, when stress and the resistance phase are prolonged, the adrenal glands can become exhausted. As you enter the exhaustion phase, your
organs or body functions begin to shut down, and you
become increasingly susceptible to illness.

STRESS AND YOUR IMMUNE SYSTEM

Your immune system, which helps protect your body against infection, is composed of the thymus, bone marrow, lymph nodes, lymphatic vessels, lymph, the liver, and the spleen. All of these components have nerve fibers that communicate with the brain. Since there is a direct link between your immune system and your mind, stress can greatly affect your body's immunity.

The thymus, the major gland of the immune system, produces T-lymphocytes. These are white blood cells that promote the cells' immunity, which is important for the body to resist infection and conditions such as allergies or cancer. The thymus also releases other hormones that regulate the functioning of the immune system.

The second major component of the immune system includes lymph, lymphatic vessels, and lymph nodes. The vessels run parallel to veins and arteries, filtering waste from body tissue and carrying lymph to the nodes. The lymph nodes filter the lymph and contain B-lymphocytes, white blood cells that promote the production of antibodies when the body is exposed to bacteria or virus.

Most of the lymph is produced by the liver. The liver contains macrophages, large cells that surround and destroy foreign substances such as bacteria, and it filters the blood. The spleen produces lymphocytes and destroys old blood cells. It also serves as a reservoir of blood that it will release in the event of hemorrhage in order to prevent your body from going into shock.

Stress has a direct adverse effect on your body's immune capacity. The immune system operates more efficiently under the parasympathetic nervous system, which controls body functions during rest and sleep. Stress, however, stimulates the sympathetic nervous system and triggers the general adaption syndrome. As your adrenal glands produce more and more hormones during stress, these chemical changes inhibit the production of white blood cells, causing the thymus to shrink. This hinders the proper functioning of the immune system—a condition known as immunosuppression—making the body more susceptible to infection and illness.

Getting Rid of Stress

Technically, "fight or flight" refers to your physiological reaction to stress, but the words also can describe how you handle stressful situations. Do you approach a conflict head-on, are you a problem-solver by nature? Or do you tend to back away from crises, letting someone else handle them instead? If you confront your problems and work them through, you probably have developed strong mechanisms or ways of coping with stress. If you avoid or ignore your problems, you are a likely candidate to develop stress-related illnesses. Do you often feel overwhelmed by a problem, unable to see your way out? Your ineffective coping mechanisms were formed long ago, but you do have the power to change them. Since stress is an inevitable part of life, you cannot do away with it completely. Natural medicine, however, can help you learn to live with stress without suffering the consequences.

Everyone's tolerance of stress is different, but when you pass your individual threshhold and stay there for a significant duration, more severe mental and physical illnesses can develop. High blood pressure, digestive conditions, headaches, insomnia, and exhaustion are major problems themselves and also can lead to deteriorated overall health. Some people seem to strive on stress, but they may not even realize the harm it is causing them until it is too late. In order to determine if you are under an inordinate amount of stress, consider whether you have trouble sleeping, nervous tics, fatigue, anxiety, or if you are easily frustrated or cry a lot for no apparent reason. If this sounds like you, you need to find a way to get rid of your excess stress.

In some circumstances stress can be positive if you can use it to face challenges productively. However, excess stress needs an outlet, such as exercise, psychotherapy, social activities, a hobby, or relaxation techniques. You should try to eliminate the cause of your stress, but if this is impossible, you need to learn to manage your reactions to it. Here are some tips for reducing your daily level of stress.

- Set limits on your workday and stick to them.
- Take breaks during the day (at least one for lunch) and try to go outside if possible—fresh air, quiet, and a walk can work wonders to soothe your nerves.
- Make exercise a regular part of your daily routine.
- Listen to soothing music whenever you feel tension begin to build.
- Eat whole (natural, unprocessed) foods and avoid sugar and caffeine.
- Practice relaxation techniques and meditation (at home and at work).

- Take a time-management and/or stress-management seminar.

- Try to pinpoint the problem(s) that is causing your stress and find a resolution.

- Confide in friends and/or see a psychotherapist or counselor—just talking about problems can help relieve some of the stress they cause.

Stress is unavoidable—everyone is affected by it at various times and in different ways. Avoiding stress will not resolve it and could have an even more debilitating influence on your mental and physical health. If you have not learned effective ways to manage stress, you might turn to ineffective or even harmful outlets. For example, some people will drink or use drugs to escape from their problems. Others might avoid the stress to the point of totally denying that they have a problem. Another person who cannot cope with stress might act out aggressively or employ one of several "defense mechanisms." One such defense mechanism is called displacement, meaning that you direct your anger or aggression toward someone "safe" rather than at the source of the stress. For instance, if your boss is giving you a hard time at work, you might go home and yell at your spouse or kids; you are displacing your anger from the source to someone who is a safe recipient of it. Another defense mechanism is called projection, the act of viewing your own problems as belonging to someone else. For example, you might blame your spouse for being overly anxious and irritable about moving when in fact you are feeling that anxiety yourself. Regression refers to the act of returning to a more childlike behavior, such as throwing a temper tantrum when things don't go your way. One of the most common defense mechanisms is rationalization, in which you "explain away" your problem or behavior. Can you recall situations in which you've used any of these defense mechanisms? While they may work to alleviate stress in the short term, they do not allow you to confront the specific conflicts and causes of the stress.

Stress takes its toll on you both physically and mentally. Natural medicine views stress as an underlying cause of all illnesses, and therefore reducing stress and learning ways to manage it are essential. The following natural medicine treatments will show you how to recognize the signs of stress, identify the causes, and learn how to live a low-stress life!

NATURAL TREATMENTS
FOR STRESS

Acupressure

Practitioners of acupressure recommend that you identify the cause of your stress, which is essential for any therapy to be truly effective. In addition to practicing acupressure, they advise creating a strategy to manage stress through exercise, meditation, and massage.

You can visit a trained acupressure practitioner if you wish, or you can apply the treatment to yourself. It is fun to learn acupressure with a friend or companion and administer treatments to each other. Having someone else apply pressure to the appropriate points allows you to totally relax your mind and body.

Before you begin, make sure that you are wearing loose, comfortable clothing—loosen your collar and belt if necessary—so that your circulation is free. If you have long nails, or if you find that your hands and fingers are not strong enough or cramp during a session, you can use a pencil eraser, golf ball, or other firm, blunt object to apply pressure on the points.

There are several ways in which you can do acupressure, and you'll need to experiment to discover what feels best. Firm pressure using fingers, palms, or knuckles means applying pressure steadily for one to several minutes. The pressure should not cause any pulling of the skin, and it should be directed at the center of the body area you are working on. Apply the pressure for one to two minutes, release and allow the tissues to respond, and then repeat. Another technique is to knead the muscles with your fingers or heels of your hands; the motion is similar to kneading dough. Rubbing an acupressure point will increase circulation, and quick tapping with your fingertips or fists stimulates the muscles.

You will experience different sensations for each point pressed, and while you may feel some soreness at particular points, you should not feel extreme pain. If pressing a particular point causes pain or a sensation in another part of your body, this "referred pain" signals that the two areas are related.

Some areas of the body can withstand greater pressure than others. For instance, the face is very sensitive, whereas the shoulders can take—and probably would enjoy—more kneading and pressure. Generally, the more developed the muscles in a given area, the more pressure they can withstand.

Acupressure is most beneficial when practiced daily, though even two or three times each week can help relieve tension and ailments. If it is feasible, do your acupressure session—limited to one hour at most—in a quiet place where you can relax totally. You can do a session at work too, as long as you can set aside ten to twenty minutes of uninterrupted time.

When you begin practicing acupressure, apply pressure for one to three minutes and gradually work up to holding points longer. You should not press a point for longer than ten minutes and should limit each area of the body to fifteen minutes. Working on a given area too long can cause too much stimulation, resulting in headache or nausea.

Stress-related tension often builds in the head, neck, shoulders, and hips. The following exercises refer to points as illustrated on pages 277–80 in the Acupressure Points section.

Head

Yintang, also called the Third Eye Point, is helpful in alleviating tension headaches and eyestrain. It is located between your eyebrows, in the indentation between the bridge of your nose and forehead. Use your middle finger to apply gentle steady pressure on the point for one minute. As you apply the pressure, focus on slow, deep breathing. Release the pressure after one minute, let your face muscles relax, and repeat the exercise.

Neck

Point GB 20 is effective for relieving tension in the neck. It is located on both sides of the body, spaced a couple of inches apart, at the base of the skull between the two vertical neck muscles. Sit comfortably and drop your head slightly. Holding the back of your head with both hands, use your thumbs to apply firm pressure to the two spots. Gently drop your head back into the pressure. When you feel a pulse on both sides, slowly release the pressure.

Shoulders

To release tension in your shoulders, press GB 21, a point located in the highest point of your shoulder muscle. Sit in a comfortable chair and allow your body to relax. Let your head drop forward, breathe deeply, and curving your fingers, apply firm pressure to GB 21 for one minute. (Caution: Pregnant women should not use this point.)

Hips

Points GB 30 and B 53, located in the pelvic area, help alleviate stress-related tensions. GB 30 is in the center of each buttock, behind the top part of the upper thighbone. B 53 is level with the second sacral hole, about three inches from either side of the spine. To use these two points, stand comfortably with your hands on your hips. Your thumbs should firmly press B 53 for one minute. Slowly release the pressure, make fists with your hands, and move them slightly down and outward to press GB30 again for one minute.

A few other points have to do with your sense of well-being. They include Lu 1, or the Central Treasury Point; CV 17, the Chest Center; and CV 12, the Center of Power. Using these points also can help you manage frustration, tension, and irritability caused by stress.

Lu 1: Central Treasury

Pressing this point will relieve chest tension and breathing problems, as well as emotional tension. It is located on the outside of the upper chest, at the level of the first intercostal space (that is, below the first rib) and six inches from the midline of the body. To use Lu 1, sit in a comfortable chair, with your back straight and head level. Use your thumbs to find the muscles at the point, and press for one minute, breathing deeply as you do so.

CV 17: Chest Center

This point is good for treating anxiety, nervousness, irritability, insomnia, and depression. It is located in the middle of the breastbone, at the level of the fourth intercostal space (that is, below the fourth rib). Use your fingers to press this point, which can be used simultaneously with Yintang (GV 24.5).

CV 12: Center of Power

To relieve emotional stress, stomach pain, indigestion, and headaches due to stress, press CV 12. It is located halfway between the base of the breastbone and navel, right in the center of the body. You can use the fingers of both hands to press this point gradually, leaning into the pressure. Apply for one minute, breathing deeply, and release. (Caution: Do not use if you have a serious illness; do not use on a full stomach, and hold no longer than two minutes.)

Aromatherapy

Many plant essences can help to bring on a calm, relaxed state of mind. Aromatherapy, or using fragrance as a natural remedy, is simple to do: Just a dip cotton in the essences and inhale. A mixture of lavender, geranium, and patchouli relieves tension and anxiety; chamomile and melissa act as antispasmodics and nerve sedatives.

To treat stress, anxiety, tension, or mental fatigue, try any one or a combination of the following: basil, bergamot, Borneo camphor, cinnamon, clove, cypress, eucalyptus, garlic, geranium, ginger, hyssop, lavender, lemon, marjoram, meroli, nutmeg, onion, peppermint, pine, rose, rosemary, thyme.

Biofeedback

Stress immediately affects your muscles by causing them to tense and tighten. This, in turn, can produce other aches and pains, such as headaches or backaches. In order to appreciate how biofeedback is effective in treating stress, it is essential to understand the role and function of muscles.

Muscles comprise the greatest mass of the body and cannot perform without nerves, which send them electrical impulses from the brain. Muscles operate on feedback systems: Nerve sensors detect their action and compare it to the preestablished notion of what that action should be. For example, when you want to write a letter, your brain directs your hand muscles to move. As they move, the nerves of your hand send information to your brain, such as what its position is and how fast it is moving. If adjustments are necessary, your brain sends messages back to your hand muscles. Of course, this complex communication between your muscles and brain occurs instantaneously.

Biofeedback operates on the notion that we have the innate ability and potential to influence the automatic functions of our bodies through the exertion of will and mind. Modern Western science tends to ignore this notion since it is not scientifically "proven" or measurable. Therefore, people generally are not taught to be aware of their internal processes and states, or to exert their mind over their body to relieve illness and maintain good health.

By helping you to become more attuned to your internal body functions, biofeedback teaches you to control certain unhealthy conditions. Muscle biofeedback equipment, for example, can measure the tension of your muscles and relay this information to you. By focusing on this information, your mind becomes less preoccupied with the problems causing stress, which in turn causes fewer messages to be sent from your brain to your muscles telling them to stay tense. You can use the information from the biofeedback instrument to make connections between the information and the way you *feel*. This increases your awareness of your own muscle tension and helps you learn to recognize tension when it first begins. Biofeedback training also teaches you ways to control the tension before other symptoms have a chance to develop.

Biofeedback machines can provide information about the systems in your body that are affected by stress. The electromyogram (EMG) measures muscle tension. Two electrodes (or sensors) are placed on your skin over the muscle to be monitored. The most common muscles that biofeedback practitioners will use are the frontalis (the "frowning" muscle in your forehead), the masseter (jaw muscle), and the trapezius (the shoulder muscles that hunch when you're stressed). When the electrodes pick up on muscle tension, the machine gives you a signal, such as a colored light or sound. In this way, you can see or hear continuous monitoring of your muscle activity and begin to focus on what the activity (or tension) *feels* like. As you become more aware of this internal process, you will begin to recognize in your daily life when tension starts to build. You then can use the techniques you learn in the biofeedback training to control the tension before it gets worse or causes other physical problems.

Another kind of biofeedback is thermograph, or temperature, training. Usually, a sensor is attached to your foot or to the middle or small finger of your dominant hand. When you are tense or anxious, your skin temperature drops as blood is redirected inward to muscles and internal organs. Like monitoring muscle tension, measuring skin temperature is a useful tool in learning how to manage stress.

Galvanic skin response (GSR) training involves monitoring the electrical conductivity of your skin. A very slight electrical current (unnoticeable to you) is run through your skin. The machine measures changes in the salt and water in your sweat gland ducts. The more emotionally aroused you are, the more active your sweat glands are and the greater the electrical conductivity of your skin. GSR is effective in treating phobias and anxiety since these emotions will affect your skin's conductivity.

Electroencephalogram (EEG) training monitors brain waves, which are classified as beta (awake), alpha (calm relaxation), theta (light sleep), and delta (deep sleep). EEG training can aid you in achieving an alpha state, though it is usually combined with other biofeedback training since an alpha state does not necessarily mean that all body systems are relaxed. EEG training also can be useful in treating insomnia.

Other biofeedback machines can monitor heart rate and blood pressure, both of which change in response to stress. You can purchase biofeedback instruments to use at home, though the most affordable are the type that monitor only one system, such as temperature. Even if you are able to invest in more expensive equipment, however, it is worthwhile to visit a trained biofeedback practitioner instead. Their professional equipment is much more accurate, and their knowledge and expertise in using the machines and administering the training is invaluable. The practitioner also will teach you relaxation techniques, and since the benefits of biofeedback are enhanced by psychotherapy, you should consider doing both simultaneously. In this way you not only learn how to control your reactions to stress but you can explore the causes of the stress and your thoughts and behavior that contribute to it.

Most large cities and universities, as well as certain hospitals, have biofeedback clinics. You can contact the Association for Applied Psychophysiology and Biofeedback (see the Natural Medicine Resources section) for a directory of certified practitioners in your area. Sessions usually last thirty to sixty minutes. The number of sessions each week and the duration of the training depend on your condition and the progress you make. The crucial last step in biofeedback training is taking what you have learned and applying it in your everyday life without the help of the machines.

Breathing Techniques

Breathing sustains life. It carries oxygen throughout the body, which purifies the blood and nourishes tissues and organs. For most of us, breathing is an involuntary, automatic process, and we are not conscious of the way we do it. You might be prone to taking short shallow breaths, or perhaps your breathing is erratic without your even knowing it. When done properly—in even, full breaths—breathing can help to counteract stress.

Before you begin to practice breathing exercises, try to become more aware of how you breathe. To do this, lie on the floor, arms and legs extended, with your eyes closed. Concentrate on your breathing, which should be through your nose. Put your hand on the spot on your chest or stomach that moves as you inhale and exhale. If this spot is on your upper chest, you are taking shallow breaths and should inhale more deeply into your lungs. Your chest and abdomen should rise and fall together with each breath. As you continue to breathe, scan your body for tense muscles and try to relax them.

Following are some breathing exercises that you can make a part of your daily relaxation routine or practice whenever you're feeling stressed out. Although you may notice benefits immediately, the long-term effect of practicing these exercises is even greater.

Complete Breathing

Find a comfortable position, either sitting or standing, and make sure that you are breathing through your nose. With each inhalation, progressively fill your lungs from the lowest point to the top: First take the air deep into your lungs so that your abdomen rises; next fill the middle of your lungs so that your ribs and chest rise; finally feel the air fill the uppermost portion of your lungs so that you draw your abdomen in slightly and your chest rises a bit. This single breath should be one continuous inhalation that takes just a few seconds.

After inhaling in this way, hold the breath for a few seconds. Exhale slowly, completely emptying your lungs, relaxing your stomach and chest.

Deep Breathing

People who tend to be nervous often take very shallow breaths, and deep-breathing exercises are especially beneficial for them. While natural breathing progressively fills your lungs, deep breathing involves inhaling into the abdomen.

Find a comfortable position, either sitting in a chair or cross-legged on the floor with your back straight or lying on the floor with your knees bent, your feet apart, and your back straight. Scan your body for tense muscles and try to relax them. Once you feel relaxed, put one hand on your stomach and one on your chest. Take a slow, deep breath in through your nose into your belly so that you feel your abdomen rise. Your chest should move slightly along with your abdomen. Since most of us are not used to breathing deeply into our abdomens, this may not feel comfortable at first. Practice this step until you do feel at ease with it before proceeding with this exercise.

Once you've mastered deep breathing, exhale by blowing out gently through your mouth. Your exhalation should sound like a soft wind. Continue to inhale long, slow deep breaths through your nose into your abdomen, and exhale through your mouth. You can practice deep breathing for five to ten minutes each day and gradually increase your time up to twenty minutes if you wish. At the end of each session, again scan your body for tension. Notice the differences in the way your body feels before and after the exercise. Deep breathing has a very calming effect and can be practiced whenever you feel tension begin to build.

Purification Breathing

This technique helps to cleanse and stimulate your lungs. Practice it when you're feeling tired or blue, and you'll feel refreshed and more alert.

Sit or stand in a comfortable position, your back straight. Inhale a complete breath (as described in the "Complete Breathing" exercise) and hold it for a few seconds. Forming a small circle with your lips, blow out just a bit of the air. Stop, and then blow out a little more. Repeat these small forceful puffs until you have completely exhaled the air. Take several breaths in this manner until you feel refreshed. You can practice this exercise alone or follow it up with another breathing exercise.

Bending Breath

This exercise is good to practice if you are feeling tense. Stand arms akimbo (hands on your hips), inhale a complete breath and hold it. Keeping the lower half of your body straight, bend forward from the waist, exhaling through your mouth. Pause and then stand up again, inhaling and holding your breath. Now bend backward as you exhale slowly through your mouth. Repeat this process bending to the left and right sides. Once you have completed a set, or round, of bending breaths, take one purifying breath, as described under "Purification Breathing," and then resume the bending breaths. Practice doing four complete rounds at a time.

Alternative Breathing

This breathing exercise, which alternates between the two nostrils, can help relieve tension and has an overall relaxing effect. To begin, sit comfortably with your back straight. Place the index and middle fingers of your right hand on your forehead, and use your thumb to close off your right nostril. Slowly inhale through your left nostril. Now close your left nostril with your ring finger while removing your thumb to open your right nostril. Slowly exhale through your right nostril. Now inhale through your right nostril, then again use your thumb to close your right nostril while opening your left nostril. Slowly exhale through the left nostril, and then inhale. Repeat this cycle five times, and gradually increase the repetitions to twenty-five times.

Exercise

When you are under stress and your body is in a fight-or-flight state, exercise is a natural way to relieve the tension. Physically, exercise improves your cardiovascular functions by strengthening and enlarging the heart, causing greater elasticity of the blood vessels, increasing oxygen throughout your body, and lowering your blood levels of fats such as cholesterol and triglycerides. All of this, of course, means less chance of developing heart conditions, strokes, or high blood pressure.

Mentally, exercise provides an outlet for negative emotions such as frustration, anger, and irritability, thereby promoting a more positive mood and outlook. Exercise also stimulates the production of neurochemicals called catecholamines into the brain and endorphins into the bloodstream. An adequate supply of catecholamines helps keep your mood stable; depressed people often lack these neurochemicals. Endorphins are natural painkillers and also help lift your mood. The runner's high you've probably heard about is a result of the increased endorphins in the body. Exercise, therefore, will keep your body functioning properly and will keep you feeling both relaxed and refreshed.

Aerobic vs. Anaerobic Exercise

There are two types of exercise that perform different functions. Aerobic exercise is sustained activity involving the major muscle groups, such as swimming, running, or brisk walking. Your heart and respiratory rate increase, and more oxygen is circulated through the body. This kind of exercise strengthens your cardiovascular system and increases your overall strength and stamina. The goal of aerobic exercise is for your pulse to reach a training rate that is appropriate for your age. You must stay at the rate for twenty minutes, and exercise three times a week, in order to reap the benefits of aerobic exercise. To determine your training heart rate, consult the chart in the section on exercise in Chapter 2.

You've probably heard of "low-impact," or anaerobic, exercise. This means that you are not exercising vigorously or long enough to reach and maintain your training heart rate. It does not mean, however, that low-impact exercise is useless. It improves your muscle strength and flexibility and can still be a good outlet for negative feelings that you might have bottled up.

There are three kinds of anaerobic exercise. Isotonics require that your muscles contract against a resistant object with movement, such as in weight lifting. Isometrics requires that your muscles contract against resistance without movement. Instead of building muscle mass, as in isotonics, isometric exercises simply increase strength without building bulk. The last group of anaerobic exercises is calisthenics. These stretching exercises, such as sit-ups, toe-touches, and knee-bends, help increase flexibility and joint mobility.

The kinds of exercises you choose to do depend on your physical ability as well as your preferences. The most important rule is to choose activities that you enjoy and that are accessible and feasible for you to do regularly. For instance, don't try to become a jogger if you really dislike running, or decide that swimming will be your exercise of choice even though you don't have reliable access to a pool. You also should consider whether you want to make your exercise routine personal time in which you can be alone with your thoughts or a more social activity. Some people find that exercising with others provides them with support and encouragement—and it can even be fun!

Before you begin an exercise program, you should have a physical examination. If you are over the age of forty, your doctor will probably want to do a stress electrocardiogram to determine how much activity your heart can handle. If you have not exercised regularly for some time, begin slowly with low-impact exercise and gradually increase your activity. If you experience any adverse side effects, such as dizziness, cramps, or chest pain, stop exercising and consult your physician.

Following is a basic low-impact exercise routine that you can do at home. Remember that this does not provide aerobic workout—for that you must choose an activity such as bicycling, running, brisk walking, swimming, aerobic dance, or use a machine such as a stationary bicycle, Lifecycle, StairMaster, or treadmill. When you exercise, wear loose, comfortable clothing and supportive sneakers.

Wait two hours after a meal before exercising in order to avoid cramping or nausea, and be sure to drink plenty of water before, during, and after your workout.

Warming Up (at least five minutes)

1. Stand with your feet a shoulder-width apart, your arms at your sides. Gently roll your head in a half circle in front of you, back and forth a few times. With your head straight, drop your left ear to your shoulder and hold. Bring your head to center and drop your right ear to your shoulder and hold. Bring your head back up and drop your chin to your chest. Head up and drop it back. Bring your head back up and face forward.

2. Shrug your shoulders up and release; repeat this six times. Roll your shoulders backward six times; roll them forward six times.

3. Place your left hand on your hip and raise your right arm up. Keeping your torso straight, reach your right arm over your head, bending to the left from your waist. Hold and then return to center. Repeat with the left arm reaching over your head to the right. You should feel a stretch in your sides.

4. Stand with your feet slightly more than a shoulder-width apart. Reach down your left leg as far as you can, trying to touch your ankle or toes if possible. Hold for ten seconds. Slowly roll yourself upright, keeping your head down to avoid dizziness. Now reach down your right leg in the same manner and hold. Again, roll up slowly with your head down. This stretches the muscles in the backs of your legs.

5. Still standing with your feet apart, turn to your left. Bend your left knee and extend your right leg straight out behind you. Center your body so that your left knee is bent at a 90-degree angle to the floor. Hold this position, called a runner's stretch, for a count of ten, gently pressing your straight leg down toward the floor. You'll feel the stretch in the thigh muscle of the out-stretched leg. Repeat this exercise with your right leg.

6. To stretch your Achilles tendon and calf muscles, stand two to three feet from a wall and place your hands on it. Keeping your legs straight and your feet flat on the floor, lean in to the wall. You should feel the stretch in your legs; hold it for ten seconds. Try stepping back a bit farther to increase the stretch; remember that your feet should remain flat on the floor.

Exercising and Conditioning (15–20 minutes)

With all of the following exercises, be sure to do the repetitions slowly and evenly, with some tension in your limbs. Your arms should not simply swing back and forth, but should move in a controlled, deliberate way, almost as if they were resisting against an invisible weight.

All of these suggest ten repetitions, but if you are just starting out, do as many as you feel comfortable doing. "No pain, no gain" may be true to some extent for accomplished athletes, but for the average person, pain often signifies stress. Try to stay tuned to the sensations in your muscles and use common sense. If it hurts too much, it's probably time to stop. As you exercise, your muscle tissue actually breaks down. In order to allow your muscles time to restore themselves, work out every other day or exercise various body areas on alternating days.

Arms

1. Stand with your feet a shoulder-width apart, stomach tucked in, and back straight. Extend your arms out to the sides with you, palms facing out. Bring your arms in together straight out in front of you, palms out, and extend back out. Do ten repetitions.

2. Keeping your arms extended, bring them straight up together above your head, then drop them so that they extend out to the sides. Repeat ten times.

3. Arms still extended with palms facing out, move your arms forward in small circles. Do ten of these and then increase to a medium-size circle. Do ten repetitions and then ten more, making the largest circle you can. Repeat this cycle, moving your arms backward.

4. Extend your arms out to the sides, bend them at the elbows, and make fists. Squeeze your bent arms together so that your forearms meet in front of you. This exercise works the chest and arms.

5. To work your biceps, extend your arms straight down at your sides with your inner forearms and fists facing up. Bending at the elbow, squeeze your fists to your shoulders. In order to obtain the maximum benefit, pretend that there is a weight on your inner forearm and resist against the pressure as you squeeze up.

Waist

1. Standing with your feet a shoulder-width apart, bend to the left, reaching slightly down and out as far as you can with your left arm. Your right hand can remain on your hip or your elbow can raise up simultaneously as you are reaching to the side with your left arm. Do ten repetitions and then repeat with the right side.

2. Standing with your feet apart, place your hands on your hips or raise your arms to chest level and bend them at the elbows so that your forearms are directly in front of your chest. Keeping your hips straight, move from the waist, twisting ten times to the left and ten times to the right. Then try alternating, pausing in the forward position between each twist.

3. This one may be a little harder to do. Sit on the floor with your legs spread open as wide as possible and your hands clasped behind your head. Keeping your back straight and your elbows back, reach down toward the floor behind your left knee with your left elbow. Come up, pause, and then reach down toward the floor with your right elbow. Do ten repetitions.

Abdomen

1. Sit on the floor with your knees slightly bent and your back straight. You can hold your arms straight out in front of you for balance, or you can cross them over your chest. From this sitting position, slowly roll back so that your shoulders are just a few inches above the floor. Pause and then slowly roll back up to a sitting position. As you do this exercise, always press the small of your back downward, rather than arching your back, in order to prevent strain. Do ten repetitions.

2. Lie on the floor with your stomach tucked in so that the small of your back presses down toward the floor. Bend your knees slightly and keep your feet flat on the floor. Clasp your hands behind your head, and, keeping your elbows back as much as possible, slowly raise your head and shoulders up off the ground. In order to help you do this exercise properly, pick a spot on the ceiling and raise your chin up toward that spot. Your head, neck, and shoulders should stay aligned and straight; you should not be "hunching" up, tucking your chin in, or using your elbows and arms to pull you up. If you don't do this exercise in the proper way, your abdomen will not benefit at all. If you do it properly, however, you will feel your abdominal muscles contract as you come up and relax as you come down. Do ten repetitions slowly and rhythmically.

3. This is a more advanced form of exercise 2. Lying in the same position, rest your left leg on your right knee. Lift your head and shoulders up in the same manner as above. Do ten repetitions and then switch legs for ten more.

Thighs

Sit on the floor with your back straight, your hands on the floor to your sides and slightly behind you with your arms straight to support your body. Keeping your right leg relaxed, straighten your left leg, point your toe, and slowly raise it up about a foot off the ground.

Lower the leg and repeat ten times. Switch legs and repeat ten times with your right leg. Remember to keep your back straight as you do this exercise.

Inner Thighs

Sitting in the same position as in the "Thighs" exercise with your legs extended straight out in front of you, lift your left leg a few inches off the floor, point your toe, and slowly move it out to the left. You'll feel a nice stretch on the inside of your thigh. Bring your leg back to the starting position, and repeat ten times. Switch legs and repeat ten times with your right leg.

Outer Thighs

Lie on your left side, your left arm bent at the elbow so that your hand supports your head, your legs stacked on top of each other. Make sure that your back is straight, and tilt your pelvis slightly toward the floor. Bend your bottom leg at the knee and keep this leg relaxed. Straighten your top leg, toe pointed, and raise it up as far as you can. You want to keep your leg straight as you raise it so that the outer thigh is parallel with the ceiling. Lower your leg and repeat ten times. When you do this exercise, pretend that there is a weight on your outer thigh and resist against it as you raise your leg. This will maximize the benefit to your muscles. Do ten repetitions and then lie on your opposite side and work your opposite leg.

Buttocks

Lie on your back, your knees bent with your feet apart, your hands clasped behind your head or placed under your buttocks. Without arching your back, lift your buttocks off the floor. Squeeze your buttocks with each lift and then release as you come back to the floor. Do ten repetitions with your feet apart and then ten with your feet together. As you master this exercise, you can do it keeping your feet apart with your knees together; with your feet together and your knees spread apart. Those who are more advanced can cross one leg over the opposite knee and vice versa.

Using the stretches described in the warm-up, be sure to spend at least five minutes cooling down after your exercise routine. If you do aerobic exercise, cool down by slowing your pace for five minutes as well as doing five minutes of stretching exercises. For example, when you're done jogging or bicycling, take a brisk walk to cool down; if you swim, cool down by doing gentle breast-, back-, or sidestrokes for five minutes. Although you may be tempted sometimes to skip the stretching, remember that your muscles have contracted and tightened during exercise, and they must be stretched out in order to prevent cramping and injuries, such as pulls.

HOMEOPATHY

Homeopathic remedies are derived from plant, animal, and mineral sources. While some of these sources are poisonous in their crude state, the remedies prepared from them are very safe and easy to use yourself. If treating yourself with homeopathy does not prove successful, or if your illness is more severe or persistent, you should consult a homeopathic health professional. If you have a basic understanding of homeopathy and want to try treating yourself, follow these guidelines. However, these treatments are not intended as a substitute for any ongoing medical treatment you may be taking. If you are under the care of a physician or are suffering from any serious illness, you should consult your doctor before undertaking any therapies.

The first thing you need to do is "take the case." When you are evaluating yourself, you must observe all symptoms, both physical and mental, as well as detailed characteristics, such as mood, speech, food cravings, effects of temperature—anything that particularly stands out. Since remedies are prescribed based on matching like with like, it is essential that you have an accurate picture of the physical and mental state of the person. Here are some things to observe as you take the case: skin, lip, and tongue color; expression and attitude; the person's body language (the way he or she moves, sits); state of mind and mood; skin temperature and sensitivity; the sound of the voice and rate of speech; pulse; breathing; description of aches and pains; times patient feels the worst; cravings or repulsions. Take notes on all of your observations and save them as health records. They might be useful in the future if illnesses recur or you notice a pattern of illnesses developing.

Once you have taken the case, you need to use the remedy that matches the symptoms most closely. This book lists the remedies that pertain to mental disorders. For a complete listing of homeopathic remedies, you need to consult a *Materia Medica*, which gives a profile of each remedy. Most books about homeopathy contain an abridged version of *Materia Medica* that lists the most widely used remedies.

You can purchase remedies from homeopathic pharmacists, and they usually come in tablet, granule, or tincture form. Tablets consist of special milk-sugar tablets that absorb the medication that is poured onto them. Granules are a powder form, and a tincture is an alcohol solution.

The standard dosage for most ailments is two tablets of a 6x potency every two to four hours. It is generally recommended that you use minimum potentizations of 6x or 12x. Of course, homeopathy respects the individuality of people and illnesses, so the dosage and intervals at which it is administered can vary depending on the person and the severity of the illness.

Remember that it is best to treat people with one remedy at a time since each pertains to a particular set of symptoms. If you use more than one at a time, discerning which effects are being caused by which remedy, and if they are contradicting each other, will be difficult. The remedies should be taken in a clean mouth that has not been subject to food, tobacco, drink, toothpaste, mouthwash, or anything else except water for at least fifteen minutes before taking the remedy. Do not take a remedy with water, but allow it to dissolve in your mouth; do not ingest anything except water for at least fifteen minutes after taking the remedy.

Continue to give the remedy until you notice improvement in the condition. At this point you can increase the intervals between doses. Once improvement is clear and persistent, you can discontinue the treatment.

It is best to store remedies in the containers they came in and to close the containers immediately after taking what you need. Make sure that the inside of the cork or cap does not come into contact with anything, and keep the containers away from heat, direct light, and pungent odors. With proper handling and storage, homeopathic remedies can last indefinitely.

The following remedies can be used to treat stress-related conditions, such as anxiety, nervousness, tension, and mental fatigue. Be sure to match your symptoms with the remedy that has the most similar characteristics.

Ignatia imara (Ignatia)

Symptoms: Emotional strain; mental stress; negative effects of grief, worry, disappointment, shock; hysteria; sad, moody, sighing; insomnia; headache, often following anger or grief, which becomes worse from stooping; intolerance to tobacco.

Worsened by: morning, suppressing emotions, tobacco, coffee, brandy, smoke or strong odors.

Better from: lying on the painful side, warmth, walking, hard pressure.

Phosphorus

Symptoms: Restlessness; overexcited state that causes weakness and exhaustion; burning pains; chilliness with thirst for cold drinks; expressive, animated, overdramatic; acute senses; bothered by light and noise; nervousness and fear; sense that something bad will happen; fearful of being alone and crave company; easily frightened or upset, though can be reassured or distracted; crave salt, spicy food, ice cream; tendency to bleed easily (this should be evaluated medically); nosebleeds.

Worsened by: cold or heat, lying on left or painful side, thunderstorms.

Better from: massaging or rubbing; cold food or drink.

HYDROTHERAPY

Hydrotherapy is safe, simple, inexpensive, and requires very little effort, yet its therapeutic benefits can be great. Most everyone has experienced the soothing or invigorating effects of a shower or bath following a long, hard day at work or intense athletic activity. No matter what is causing the stress in your life, hydrotherapy can help to ease the tension.

Generally, heat quiets and soothes the body, slowing down the activity of internal organs. Cold, in contrast, stimulates and invigorates, increasing internal activity. If you are experiencing tense muscles and anxiety from your stress, a hot shower or bath is in order. If you are feeling tired and stressed out, you might want to try taking a warm shower or bath followed by a short, invigorating cold shower to help stimulate your body and mind. Experiment with different water temperatures and durations in the bath or shower to determine what water method works best for you. Remember, the goal is to use hydrotherapy to achieve a state of comfort, relaxation, and refreshment.

Herbal baths can be particularly soothing when you are experiencing a period of stress. There are several ways to prepare an herbal bath:

1. Simmer ½ cup of herbs in 1 quart of water in a covered pot for fifteen minutes. While the herbs are simmering, take a short shower to cleanse your body, then fill the tub with hot or warm water. Strain the liquid from the decoction into the bath water, and wrap the herbs in a washcloth. Soak in the tub for at least twenty minutes, using the "herbal washcloth" to rub over your body.

2. Add ½ cup of herbs to running bath water, preferably hot. You might want to cover the drain with a thin mesh screen to prevent the herbs from clogging the pipes. Soak in the tub for twenty to thirty minutes.

3. Fill a thin cloth bag with ½ cup of herbs, either placing it in the bath water or tying it to the spigot so that the hot water runs through it as it fills the tub. Again, soak for twenty to thirty minutes.

Certain herbs are quite effective for creating soothing baths. Combine a handful each of valerian, lavender, linden, chamomile, hops, and burdock root, and add it to your bath according to one of the preceding methods. Soak for thirty minutes in the tub. Another soothing herbal bath calls for a handful each of hops, linden, valerian, chamomile, yarrow, and passionflower. Prepare this bath according to one of the preceding methods, or simmer the herbs in a quart of water, then drink ½ cup of the liquid (with lemon and honey added, if you wish) and pour the rest in the tub. While soaking in an herbal bath, you can read, meditate, listen to peaceful music, or just sit quietly, concentrating on relaxing yourself.

NUTRITION

Balanced nutrition is essential to maintaining overall good health, but it also can affect your capacity to cope with stress. When you are going through a period of stress, you need more of all nutrients, particularly the B vitamins, which affect the nervous system, and calcium, which is needed to counteract the lactic acid your tense muscles produce. Likewise, if you are lacking nutrients, your body will not be equipped to handle stress effectively.

It is most important to eat a variety of foods to ensure that you consume all of the forty to sixty nutrients you need to stay healthy. These include vitamins, minerals, amino acids (from proteins), essential fatty acids (from vegetable oil and animal fat), and energy from carbohydrates, protein, and fat. While most foods contain more than one nutrient, no single food provides adequate amounts of all nutrients. You should eat the following number of servings from the basic food groups each day.

Vegetables:	3–5 (serving = ½ cup)
Fruit:	2–4 (serving = ½ cup or 1 piece of fruit)
Bread, cereals, grains:	6–11 (serving = 1 slice or ¾ cup cereal)
Dairy products:	2–3; 3–4 for teens, pregnant or nursing women (serving = 1 cup milk or yogurt, 1 slice cheese)
Meat, poultry, fish, eggs, legumes:	2–3 (serving = 3 ounces lean meat; 2 eggs; 1¼ cups legumes)

Try to maintain a diet of mostly whole (unprocessed) foods, as they contain the most nutrients and are not contaminated with additives, which can be harmful or cause allergic reactions. Stay away from caffeine (coffee, tea, cola, chocolate), which causes nervousness and inhibits sleep if too much is ingested. Caffeine causes a fight-or-flight response in your body and uses up your reserves of the B vitamins, which are important in coping with stress. Alcohol also depletes your body's B vitamins, and can disrupt sleep and impair your judgment or clarity of thought. Avoid sugar too, which provides no essential nutrients and can cause an immediate "high" followed by a prolonged "low."

Studies have shown that the body depletes its stores of nutrients when under stress, mainly protein and the B vitamins as well as vitamins C and A. A deficiency of magnesium, which helps muscles relax, has been linked to

"Type A" or high-stress personalities. If you are under prolonged stress or are at risk for hypertension, consume foods high in potassium, such as orange juice, squash, potatoes, apricots, limes, bananas, avocados, tomatoes, and peaches. You also should increase your intake of calcium, which is found in yogurt, cheese, tofu, and chickpeas.

If you eat balanced meals, taking supplements usually is not necessary. The following chart illustrates the nutrients that are essential to proper functioning of the nervous system, their natural sources, the recommended daily allowance (RDA) to prevent disease, and the recommended daily dose (RDD) you need to maintain optimal health.

Vitamin/Minerals	*Source*	*RDA*	*RDD*
Vitamin A	green vegetables, milk, liver, kidney, fish liver oil	5,000 i.u.	—
Vitamin B^1 (Thiamine)	yeast, kelp, wheat germ, milk, green vegetables, meat, liver, oysters	1.5 mg	75 mg
Vitamin B^2 (Riboflavin)	yeast, wheat germ, soybeans, peanuts, green vegetables, milk, eggs, meat, poultry	1.7 mg	75 mg

Vitamin/Minerals	Source	RDA	RDD
Vitamin B^3	yeast, liver, eggs, bran, brown rice	20 mg	75 mg
Vitamin B^6	yeast, wheat germ, milk, fish, melon, cabbage, egg yolk	2 mg	200 mg
Vitamin B^{12}	yeast, spinach, eggs lettuce, liver, meat	6 mcg	75 mg
Vitamin C	citrus fruit, tomatoes, raw vegetables, melon	60 mg	2–10 g
Vitamin D	milk, butter, eggs, fish liver oil, green vegetables	400 units	800 units
Vitamin E	egg yolks, milk, seed germ oils, green vegetables	30 i.u.	400 i.u.
Biotin	kidney, liver, nuts, vegetables	150 mcg	150 mcg
Calcium	dairy products, bone meal, calcium lactate	1000 mg	3 g
Folic acid	green leafy vegetables liver, brewer's yeast	400 mcg	400 mcg

Vitamin/Minerals	Source	RDA	RDD
Iodine	plant and animal seafoods	160 mcg	40 mg
Magnesium	green vegetables, corn, apples, almonds, soybeans	350 mg	1.5 g
Potassium	leafy vegetables, whole grains, oranges, potato skins	none	2 g

If you find that you have difficulty managing stress and often feel fatigued or stressed out, you might want to examine your diet for deficiencies in certain nutrients. You can do this yourself by keeping meticulous records of everything you eat, broken down into specific nutrients; or you can seek the help of a physician or nutritionist who can provide an accurate assessment of your dietary needs. If you are deficient in certain nutrients, particularly any of those just mentioned, you will need to alter your diet or perhaps even take supplements.

Since every person is unique, nutritional needs vary to some degree. It will probably take several months to change your diet and establish healthy eating habits, but be patient! Experimenting and taking the time to reform your eating will have very positive immediate and long-term effects. Choose foods that you enjoy and try to make meals pleasurable times. You may think eating on the run now and then is unavoidable, but if you work on managing your time—and your stress—you will find that it is possible, and even desirable, to set aside as little as ten to fifteen minutes for eating a relaxed meal. Continue your healthy diet and supplements even after the period of stress has passed so that your body will be best prepared to cope with the next stressful situation you encounter. The goal is to maintain maximum health with good nutrition, exercise, and active stress management.

RELAXATION TECHNIQUES

Meditation

Relaxation exercises are an important component of biofeedback, but they also are good therapy as well. One popular method of relaxation is meditation. There are many different kinds of meditation, but one approach involves clearing your mind of all thoughts to achieve a heightened state of awareness. This may seem impossible, and probably will be at first. Your mind most likely will race with thoughts—what to cook for dinner, when to pick up the children, that deadline for your annual report at work, the phone calls you need to make. With regular practice, though, you may be able to quiet your mind and become more attuned to yourself.

Although there are different meditation techniques, it is common to sit quietly, either in a chair or cross-legged on the floor, keeping your back straight and your hands resting on your knees. If it is more comfortable, you also can practice meditation lying down, though most schools of meditation recommend a sitting position. Close your eyes and allow yourself to become aware of yourself.

Think about the way you are sitting, the way the floor or chair feels, the sensations at the points where your body touches itself. Centering yourself for meditation begins with an awareness of yourself physically in the moment and also involves your breathing.

Let your breathing be steady, deep, and rhythmic. Inhale deeply to a slow count of two, and exhale slowly to the count of four. Concentrate on the flow of your breath in and out of your body. Feel where the air goes and how it moves. Inhale into your chest, then stomach, then deep into your lower abdomen. Your abdomen should expand and deflate as air goes in and out. This is the most relaxing way to breathe for meditation. If it feels forced or uncomfortable at first, keep at it—it will become natural over time.

Some people like to chant a mantra or repeat a specific phrase over and over. Your mantra can be as simple as a single word, such as "calm" or "one." Chanting while you meditate has a somewhat hypnotic effect and can enhance the effects of the meditation. Gazing at a soothing object, such as flowers or a candle flame, can have the same effect. If you can achieve a meditative state, your body will totally relax and you will increase your sense of self-awareness.

Although some people have been skeptical about meditation, scientific evidence supporting its effects has been available for years. In 1968, researchers at Harvard Medical School tested meditators to see what effects meditation had on the body. They found that, during meditation, the body processes are the opposite of what they are during their reaction to stress. Therefore, meditation is a valuable exercise to help you overcome stress and tension.

Following are some meditation variations that you can practice. You might find that particular ones work better for you than others, or that you enjoy alternating them each time you meditate. Whichever exercises you do, remember that consistent practice is needed to receive the maximum benefit from meditation.

Observing Your Thoughts and Letting Them Go

In this form of meditation, you do not rid your mind of thoughts, but note them and let them go. To begin, choose a comfortable, quiet place, close your eyes, and center yourself. As a thought or feeling passes through your mind, observe it and then simply let it go. It might help to imagine your thoughts and feelings as elusive objects that appear and then disappear, such as bubbles that rise to the surface of a pond and then pop, or a bird that flies overhead and then is gone. For example, if the thought of doing your laundry enters your mind, imagine this thought to be a bubble rising to the surface; watch it rise, and then watch it pop. You should simply observe your thoughts but not dwell on them. Just let them go.

Gazing Meditation

In this meditation exercise, you focus your stare on a particular object, but do not think about that object in words. Begin by choosing an object that you like. It can be anything from a seashell or wooden sculpture, to the clouds or a favorite tree. Once you have your object before you, sit in a comfortable posture, center yourself, and fix your gaze on the object. Observe the object as if this is the first time you are seeing it; take in its size, color, and texture, moving your eyes over the entire object as it is visible to you. Try not to think about the object in words, not to analyze or judge it, but to experience its various qualities. When words or thoughts do come up, observe them and let them go.

Meditation for Tension Release

Meditation is an excellent way for you to become more aware of muscle tension. To begin, find a comfortable posture, center yourself, and breathe deeply. Start with your head and focus your attention there. Take note of all sensations in that area: Is your forehead furrowed, do your eye muscles ache, are your lips pressed together tightly, are you clenching your jaw? After you focus for a moment on each of these sensations in your head, move your attention to your neck, and concentrate on what that area feels like. If you feel tension in any body part or area, try to relax those muscles and let the tension flow out of your body. Continue in this way, moving down your body to each body part, focusing on the sensations there and letting go of the tension.

Meditation for Relief of Discomfort and Pain

People have come to rely on aspirin and other painkillers to relieve discomforts, aches, and pains. An alternative way of coping with pain is not to try to get rid of it, because often this is impossible, but to allow yourself to experience it. Usually when we feel an irritation or pain, the muscles in that general area will tighten in response to it, and the tension adds to the discomfort. This meditation exercise can help you to learn to relax the area around the point of discomfort in order to focus just on the painful point itself.

First find your posture, center yourself, and breathe deeply. Throughout the meditation, try not to move at all; if you do, just observe your movement and then return your concentration to the meditation. Soon you will begin to realize when you are about to move before you actually do it. Once you have achieved this level of awareness, try to focus on why you want to move—is it because you have an itch or an aching back? Whatever the irritation is, notice whether the muscles in that area are tensing up and try to relax them. Concentrate on the discomfort itself and what it feels like. At the end of your meditation, you can shift your position or move the way you had wanted to move. As you do, notice the feeling—is it relief? Does this make your body more comfortable? If you still feel any tension, try to let it go.

Meditate While Walking

Many of us bustle around each day, not taking time to appreciate our environment or notice how the frenzied pace is making us feel physically and emotionally. Meditating while you walk can help solve both of these problems. As you begin your walk (either around the block or a park, or to the bus stop or your office), concentrate on breathing from your abdomen, taking the air deep into your belly and releasing it from the same spot. Now begin counting the number of steps you take as you inhale and the number as you exhale: for example, in—two—three, out—two—three—four. Your steps need not be uniform, but can change with each breath; the consistency is not important, but the concentration on the actions of walking and breathing is.

In another kind of walking meditation, you can focus your attention on the experience of walking. How do your legs and feet feel? Which muscles can you feel working? What is the movement of your knees? How does the ground feel beneath your feet? Observe the lay of the land, the textures and colors of grass, dirt, pavement, leaves, rocks. Simply observe all of these things and then let them go.

Eating Meditation

This meditation is similar to the walking exercises. Most of us don't take much time out for meals, unless they are marking special occasions. Fast food has certainly helped fuel our ability to eat on the run, and this can cause heartburn and indigestion and worsen already existing stress. Try to set aside time at certain meals to meditate while you eat. Begin by sitting comfortably and taking several deep breaths. Gaze for a moment at your food and note your reaction to it—are you starving and ready to devour it, or do you feel indifferent toward it? When you are ready to begin eating, take note of your movements: your hand lifting your fork, spearing your food, raising it to your mouth. Repeating to yourself what you are doing—lifting, spearing, raising, and so on—might help you to stay focused on your actions. Again notice your body's reactions as you get ready to take a bite; your mouth may begin to water or your stomach start to growl. As you eat, again focus on each action: biting, chewing, the movement of the food in your mouth, swallowing. Follow the movement of the food from your mouth into your esophagus, and note any sensation you may feel in your stomach. As you continue to eat, keep concentrating on all of your movements and sensations.

As you probably have gathered, the goal of meditation is to increase your awareness of ordinary experiences. This, in turn, will heighten your awareness and understanding of yourself—your thoughts, your feelings, and your sensations. Sometimes, as your mind becomes increasingly clear and calm with meditation, unconscious feelings, such as fear or anger, that you have repressed might come to the surface. If this happens to you, try to allow yourself to have the feelings without analyzing them during your meditation. If the feelings persist and you feel the need to talk about them, by all means seek out a friend or counselor.

Progressive Relaxation

Progressive relaxation was developed in the 1920s by Dr. Edmund Jacobson, a physician in Chicago. The technique is also referred to as "tense-relax" exercises, as this is exactly what the activity entails: You successively tense and then relax various groups of muscles. When you begin a stress-management program or routine, progressive relaxation is a good starting point because it helps you to identify where all of your muscles are located. It gives you a greater overall awareness of your body and where your tension lies.

Some people are so accustomed to being tense that they don't even recognize the sensations of tension. For instance, do you find that your neck and shoulders automatically tense up when you begin to drive? Or at work, does your hand clench the phone whenever you pick it up? Often, in our efforts to deflect or deal with everyday stressors, our bodies respond with tension almost instinctively. And when this happens enough, it begins to feel normal.

Using progressive relaxation to enhance your awareness of your muscles also will increase your sensitivity to the difference between feeling tense and feeling relaxed. Then, when you feel tension beginning to build, you can employ exercises to help stave it off before it worsens and causes other physical symptoms, such as headaches, nausea, or pain. Physically, progressive relaxation helps to decrease your blood pressure, pulse rate, and respiration rate. It is beneficial in treating muscular tension, anxiety, depression, and fatigue, among other ailments.

In order to achieve maximum results, try to make progressive relaxation sessions part of your daily routine. Set aside fifteen to thirty minutes, depending on your schedule and needs, twice each day. Find a quiet place to practice—if not at home, perhaps at the local library or a park. If you want to practice at work, do so on a break or during your lunch hour. Some people find that it is useful to do just a few minutes of progressive relaxation at the moment when they first detect tension starting to build. Whatever routine works best for you, be sure to choose times and places that will be most conducive to your practicing every day.

Progressive Relaxation Exercise

Find a comfortable position, either lying flat on your back or sitting in a comfortable chair. Loosen any restrictive clothing or shoes so that you are not distracted or uncomfortable. Beginning with one area of your body—your arm, for instance—you will tense each part—for example, first your fists, then your forearms, biceps, and so on. After holding and concentrating on the tension for approximately five seconds, you release it and relax that body part for about twenty seconds. It might help you to relax if you instruct yourself with a phrase such as "Relax and let go" or "Let the tension go." Once you finish with a specific area, move on to the next region. You should repeat the tense/relax exercise at least once with each body part, though you can tense and relax each up to five times, depending on what feels comfortable and effective to you. During the progressive relaxation procedure, you want to continually take note of the difference in the sensations of tension and relaxation.

You can practice the progressive relaxation exercise by mentally going through each body region, or you can make a tape recording that leads you through the exercise. If you do make a tape, remember to speak slowly and to pause long enough after each instruction to allow for the action to occur. Following is an example of a procedure that you can record.

Let your body relax, feel the tension flow out of your body. Make a fist with your right hand and squeeze, feeling the muscles tighten. Concentrate on the tension in your fist, and note the tension spreading to your forearm. Now open your fist and relax your hand. Let it dangle and hang limp; notice the difference between how it feels now and how it felt when it was tensed. Now do the same with your left hand: Make a fist and clench it. Feel the tension spreading up your arm. Now let the fist hang loose, and again, feel the difference.

Let's move to the upper arm. Bend your right arm at the elbow and squeeze your biceps as hard as you can. Focus on the tension and how it feels. Now relax your arm and let go of the tension; notice the difference between the tensed biceps and the relaxed one. Repeat this step with your left biceps. When you are done, relax both of your arms. Feel the tension flow out of your arms and deep relaxation set in.

Next move to your neck and shoulders. Hunch your shoulders forward and feel the tension; now let them relax. Starting at the left, gently roll your neck down and forward and around to the right, then slowly roll it back to the left. Repeat the half roll and feel the stretching sensation move from the muscles in the side of your neck, to those in back, to those on the opposite side. Now drop your left ear toward your shoulder and feel the muscles stretching on the right side of your neck. Return your head to its natural position and take a deep breath. Then drop your right ear toward your shoulder and feel the muscles stretching on the left side of your neck. Again return your head to its natural position and take a deep breath. Now drop your head forward and press your chin to your chest; feel the muscles in the back of your neck stretch. Drop your head back and feel the tension in your throat and back of your neck. Now bring your head forward to rest in a natural position. Feel the tension flow out of your neck. Check your shoulders and make sure that they are not tensed. If they are, drop them and let them relax. Feel the tension go away; feel the relaxation getting deeper.

Now move to your head. Clench your jaw and feel the tension in your jaw and cheeks. Relax your jaw and feel the tension dissolve. Now open your mouth as wide as you can. Again feel the face muscles pull. Now close your mouth and relax your face. The tension is gone and you are calm and relaxed. Next focus on your eyes. Squeeze them shut, feeling the face muscle straining. Relax your face and keep your eyes closed gently. Furrow your brow as hard as you can and feel the muscles in your forehead tense. Relax your brow and forehead and let the tension go. Notice the difference between feeling tense and feeling relaxed. Take a deep breath and slowly exhale. Feel the tension flow away from your face and head. The relaxation is going deeper and deeper.

Now move down to your chest. Take a deep breath in, filling your lungs. Hold your breath and feel the tension in your ribs. Slowly exhale and notice how the tension slips away. Repeat this procedure, and then pause to take a few normal, gentle breaths. Next take a deep breath, inhaling into your stomach. Feel your stomach fill with air like a balloon; hold the breath there, feeling the tautness of your stomach. Slowly release the breath and feel the tension blow away. Next squeeze your stomach muscles in as tight as you can. Hold the tension and then release, feeling your stomach muscles relax. Note the difference between the tension and the relaxation that replaces it.

You are now feeling more relaxed and calm. Your stomach is relaxed, your chest is relaxed . . . your shoulders are dropped and relaxed . . . your head rests comfortably on your neck and both are relaxed . . . your arms are dangling or resting comfortably . . . there is no tension now. Your entire upper body is deeply relaxed.

Now focus your attention on your lower body. Squeeze your buttocks and hold the tension. Then let it go and feel your buttocks relax. Keeping the rest of your body relaxed, tense your thigh muscles. Hold it briefly and then let your thighs relax. Next squeeze your calf muscles and concentrate on the tension. Now relax your calves and let the relaxation replace the tension. Notice the difference between the two. Finally, curl your toes and squeeze. Feel the tension in your feet and spreading into your legs. Uncurl your toes and relax your feet. Now raise your toes up and feel the tension on the tops of your feet and in your shins. Release your toes and let your feet relax. Let the tension flow out of them as your entire body becomes totally, deeply relaxed.

You have moved through all of your major muscles, tensing and releasing, allowing the relaxation to replace the tension. Now tense your entire body, every muscle you can possibly muster. Hold the tension briefly, then relax and let the tension go. Your muscles will soften and smooth out; the tension is flowing out of your body. Take a deep breath in and exhale. Continue breathing steadily, deeply; each time you exhale, imagine that tension is leaving your body. You become more and more relaxed with every breath you take.

Autogenic Training

Autogenic, which means "self-regulation or -generation," refers to the way in which your mind can influence your body to balance the self-regulative systems that control circulation, breathing, heart rate, and so on. Autogenic training allows you to control stress by training your autonomic nervous system to become relaxed.

Since autogenic training does not involve direct muscle relaxation, it is best to learn progressive relaxation first. Autogenic training will then teach you to respond, in a passive rather than active manner, to verbal and visual cues that reduce tension. By focusing on relaxing phrases and images, the training conditions positive, relaxing responses, such as rhythmic breathing and heart rate and a warm, relaxed, heavy feeling throughout the body.

Autogenic training is based on the notion of passive concentration: that is, you try to achieve your goal of relaxation by *not* working actively to do so (as in progressive relaxation). For example, instead of instructing yourself, "Your heart beat will slow down," you focus on a phrase, such as "My heart is beating gently and evenly," or an image, such as ripples in a pond to induce the response of relaxation.

Similar to progressive relaxation, you should practice autogenic training twice each day in order to maximize the benefits. Again, choose times and places that are feasible for an uninterrupted session. Your clothes should be comfortable, and you should sit or lie in a position that allows total support for your entire body. When you begin autogenic training, first work on reducing your heart rate and calming your breathing; then you can move on to trying to evoke warm, heavy, relaxed sensations in your limbs and body.

As you practice, try to combine phrases with images in order to keep your mind occupied. If thoughts do intrude into your session, just observe them and let them go. Following is an example of a session using phrases and images. You can run through this mentally as you practice, or you can make a tape recording to guide you through the session.

Sit comfortably and gently roll your head in a half circle in front of you. Roll from side to side a few times then bring your head up to face forward. Take a deep breath in, drawing the air deep into your stomach. Slowly release the breath.

Concentrate on your breathing, which is smooth and rhythmic. Imagine that your breaths are like waves lapping at the shore. Keep this image in your mind as you repeat to yourself, "My breathing is rhythmic and smooth . . . my breathing is rhythmic and smooth."

With each breath, feel relaxation wash over you like the waves. The waves wash over your feet and legs, your stomach and chest. Feel them cover your arms, your neck, your head. Your arms and legs feel warm and heavy. Feel the waves of relaxation sweep over you. Feel your limbs growing heavier, warmer. Your breathing is calm, rhythmic, and smooth.

Now move your focus to your heart. Imagine the waves of relaxation washing over you, calming your breathing and your heart. Say to yourself, "My heartbeat is gentle and even . . . my heartbeat is gentle and even." "I feel quiet, calm, relaxed . . . my heartbeat is gentle and even."

Your body feels peaceful and tranquil, you are relaxed. Concentrate now on your right arm and hand. Say to yourself, "My right arm and hand feel warm and heavy . . . my right arm and hand feel warm and heavy." Imagine the sun shining on your arm and hand. Feel the warmth spread through your arm and hand as they grow heavier and heavier. Say to yourself, "My right arm and hand feel warm and heavy . . ."

Now focus on your left arm and hand. Say to yourself, "My left arm and hand feel warm and heavy . . . my left arm and hand feel warm and heavy." Again imagine the sun shining on your arm and hand, or that they are soaking in a hot tub. Feel the warmth spread through your arm and hand, and feel them grow heavier. Say to yourself, "My left arm and hand feel warm and heavy . . ."

Concentrate now on both of your arms and hands. They both feel warm and heavy. Say to yourself, "Both of my arms and hands are warm and heavy . . . my right arm and left arm are warm and heavy . . ." Feel the warmth flow through your arms and hands, down into your fingers to the tips. You feel relaxed all over as your arms and hands get warmer and heavier. While your arms are warm and heavy, scan your body from head to toe to find any muscle tension in other parts of your body. Make sure your shoulders are dropped and relaxed, your jaw is not clenched, your legs are relaxed. You should feel relaxed all over, your mind free from thought.

Now turn your concentration to your legs. Feel the warmth and heaviness from your arms flow down into your legs. Say to yourself, "My legs and feet are warm and heavy . . . my legs and feet are warm and heavy." Imagine bathing in the sun and feel the warmth spread over your body, radiating through your arms and hands, down through your legs and feet. Say to yourself, "My feet and hands are warm and heavy . . . my arms and legs are warm and heavy." All of your limbs now feel warm and heavy. Your body is relaxed and calm, your breathing is deep and rhythmic, your heart is beating gently and evenly.

To complete the autogenic exercise, take a deep breath and exhale. Picture yourself now in the room where you began the session. You are calm and relaxed, and you will become more relaxed each time you do this exercise. Take a few more deep breaths, open your eyes, and you will feel relaxed yet alert and refreshed.

If you are going to resume physical activity, you can follow your autogenic exercises with stretching to stimulate your muscles. If you find yourself yawning, don't assume that you are now tired. Take this as a sign that the exercise has worked—that you are relaxed and free from tension.

While autogenic training is effective in reducing stress, tension, and anxiety, it is not recommended for people with severe mental disorders. You should have a complete physical examination before beginning to practice autogenic training, and people with diabetes, hypoglycemia, heart conditions, and high or low blood pressure should practice only under the supervision of their physician. If you feel any adverse side effects, discontinue your practice and consult with an experienced autogenic training instructor.

Imagery Training or Visualization

You've probably heard the expression You are what you think you are. In other words, your thoughts have a direct influence on the way you feel and behave. For instance, if you tend to dwell on sad or negative thoughts, you most likely are not a very happy person. Likewise, if you think that your job is enough to give you a headache, you probably will come home with throbbing temples each day. This is just another clear example of the power the mind exerts over the body.

Your imagination can be a powerful tool to help you combat stress, tension, and anxiety. You can use visualization to harness the energy of your imagination, and it does not take long—probably just a few weeks—to master the technique. Try to visualize two or three times a day. Most people find it easiest to do in bed in the morning and at night before falling asleep, though with practice you'll be able to visualize whenever and wherever the need arises.

To begin visualization, sit or lie down in a comfortable position and close your eyes. Scan your body for any muscle tension and relax the areas that need it. Once you feel relaxed, begin to visualize a scene, object, or place that is soothing and pleasing to you. Imagine every aspect of the scene, involving all of your senses. For example, if you like to visualize a waterfall on a mountain, imagine first what this looks like: the rushing water, the stream flowing from it, the size and thickness of the trees all around, the sky above and the sun filtering through the branches, and so on. Then imagine how this place would smell—damp and musty or fragrant pine. Next listen for the sounds you would hear if you were there: the water rushing over rocks, the hush of the wind rising and then quieting down, birds singing and crickets chirping. How does the ground feel beneath your feet? Is it rocky and rough, or soft and smooth from pine needles or moss? Imagine chewing on a blade of grass, or taking a long, cool drink from the waterfall. How do these taste?

As you become more involved in your visual image, your body will relax and you will be able to let go of the problems or worries that you'd felt before. To encourage this relaxation to occur, you can punctuate the images with positive statements, such as "I am letting go of tension" or "I feel calm and relaxed." Using the subject of your favorite place, here is an example of a visualization exercise that you can tape record. If you do record it, or something similar to this, be sure to speak slowly and allow generous pauses so your visualizations can form.

Sit or lie down, close your eyes, and take deep breaths. Scan your body for tension and try to relax those muscles. (long pause) Once your body feels relaxed, go to your favorite place . . . it is calm and safe, a place where your worries disappear. Look around at this place and take in all the sights. How does it feel to be here? You are safe and at peace. Notice what you hear in this special place. What do you smell? Walk a bit farther into your favorite place. Look up, and down, and all around. Notice what you see and how it makes you feel. Say to yourself, "I am relaxed . . . my worries are gone . . . tension has flowed out of my body." Take in all of the sights, sounds, smells, and feelings of this special place. You can return here whenever your want to. Repeat to

yourself, "I am relaxed here . . . this is my favorite
place."

When you have thoroughly visualized this place,
open your eyes but stay in the same comfortable position. Continue to breathe smoothly and rhythmically,
and take a few moments to experience and enjoy your
relaxation. Rest assured that your special place is available to you whenever you need to go there.

Another type of visualization involves an image that
you associate with tension which you can replace with an
image for relaxation. For example, you might visualize
tension as a taut rope, the sound of thunder, the color red,
pitch darkness, persistent hammering, or blinding white
light. These images of tension can soften and fade into
images of relaxation. For instance, the taut rope loosens,
the thunder subsides and is replaced by a light rain, red
turns to orchid, the darkness begins to lighten, the pounding hammer is replaced by the murmur of cicadas and
crickets, the blinding white light softens to a sunset.

When you feel a muscle becoming tense, imagine that
it is one of these tension images. Then let it transform
into a relaxation image as you repeat to yourself, "I can
relax . . . the tension is slipping away."

It has been suggested that you can make tape recordings, following the examples given in this book, to guide
you through your relaxation exercises. There are also
many good tapes available on the market. New Harbinger
Publications produces *Body Awareness and Imagination*,
about visualization and scanning your body for tension;
Autogenics and Meditation, a basic twelve-week program

in autogenics techniques, breathing, and meditation; and *Progressive Relaxation and Breathing,* for relaxing muscles and reducing tension. You can order these tapes, currently priced at $11.95 each, by calling 1-800-748-6273. Stress Management Research Associates, Inc., located at P.O. Box 2232-B, Houston, Texas 77251, offers a cassette and guidebook program for stress management. The tapes include *Progressive Relaxation and Deep Muscle Relaxation, Autogenic Relaxation: Arms & Hands and Legs & Feet, Visual Imagery Relaxation and Image Rehearsal Practice.* The entire package is currently $34.95 (plus $1.50 postage), or cassettes can be purchased individually for $12.95 each.

Music is also useful in the practice of relaxation and stress management as it can evoke pleasing and soothing sensations to the listener. Epic Records has produced meditative selections by Paul Horn called *Inside (The Taj Mahal)* and *Inside 2.* Tony Scott's *Music for Zen Meditation* and *Tibetan Bells* is available from Verve. Atlantic Records puts out a series of recordings of environmental sounds called *Environments.* New Age and classical music is also pleasing to listen to, though your selections will of course be a matter of personal taste and preference.

By now you probably have a better understanding of the role stress plays in your life. While moderate occasional stress is inevitable, chronic stress can be harmful to your physical and mental health. But no matter how often, how intense, or for how long you experience stress, there are many natural medicine remedies and treatments that can help you cope with the difficult times and manage stress on a daily basis.

CHAPTER FIVE

Anxiety Disorders: Feeling Like a Twisted Rope

All people, at times, experience "raw nerves" or find themselves in circumstances that make them feel nervous and apprehensive. Appropriately, the Latin root of the word "anxiety" means "twisted rope," and this pretty much describes how you feel when you have an attack of anxiety. Usually anxiety can be controlled to some degree and will pass when the situation changes or the stressor is removed. But when does ordinary anxiety reach the point of being diagnosed as a disorder?

Anxiety is considered an illness when you cannot control your anxious feelings. Anxiety disorders involve excessive levels of negative emotions, such as fear, worry, nervousness, and tension, and the anxious feelings occur involuntarily despite your best attempts to avoid them or stave them off.

There are basically two types of anxiety. Exogenous anxiety, which is provoked by an identifiable danger or stressor existing outside of the person, is a normal reaction. For instance, if your child is ill with a high fever, your exogenous anxiety is a natural response to the situation. Endogenous anxiety, produced within the person, can be caused by internal conflicts, such as having to make a tough decision. With endogenous anxiety, the cause of the anxious feelings is not always identifiable. Sometimes symptoms of anxiety come on suddenly, with no apparent reason, and cause you to feel as if you're not in control of your body. This kind of endogenous anxiety may be diagnosed as anxiety disorder. While medications can help alleviate the symptoms in extreme cases, natural medicine treatments also are effective in managing the anxiety and preventing it from recurring.

CAUSES OF ANXIETY DISORDERS

As with most mental disorders, it is difficult to pinpoint an exact cause of anxiety disorder. Rather, it is brought about by the interplay of biological, psychological, and environmental factors. The biological component refers to the chemical composition of the body, which might be off balance. Psychological factors have to do with the behaviors and attitudes you have learned throughout your life. Environmental factors refer to external stressors, the conflicts, problems, and pressures you must deal with.

Studies show that there is a biological component to anxiety disorders and that the susceptibility to developing them is genetically inherited to some extent. If you have a close relative who has anxiety disorder, you are more likely to develop the disorder than those who do not; the closer the relative is, the more likely you are to develop it. Studies done on twins show that identical twins are more likely to share the disorder than nonidentical twins. This finding suggests that the genetic inheritance, or biological factors, outweighs the environmental causes.

Research points to a chemical imbalance in the body as causing the symptoms of anxiety disorder. One theory suggests that certain nerve endings and receptors in the central nervous system overwork, producing too much catecholamines, the stimulants that excite the brain. At the same time, there may be a deficiency in the neurotransmitters that inhibit the stimulation of the brain. The overabundance of catecholamines and lack of inhibitory neurotransmitters combine to cause the symptoms of anxiety.

Psychological factors, or the way you have been taught to think, can influence whether you develop an anxiety disorder. For example, if either or both of your parents were constant worriers, chances are that you might be a nervous, worrying personality too. Were you raised in a family that wouldn't allow you to touch dogs and cats because they were seen as dirty? If so, you might develop a strong aversion to either of these animals. Of course, it's not a given that certain conditions will automatically or definitely cause the development of an anxiety disorder. However, they can contribute to the possibility that you will develop one.

Anxiety disorders can be fostered by classical conditioning, a psychological term that refers to the association of one thing with another. You've probably heard of Pavlov's dogs. Pavlov was a scientist who trained dogs to associate the sound of bells with food. He found that even when there was no food, the sound of the bells would stimulate the dogs, by association, to begin salivating in anticipation of food. Similarly, a person may learn to associate anxiety with a particular situation, place, or object. For example, if you had an anxiety attack while shopping in a crowded store, the connection between the anxiety and crowds (or stores) becomes solidified in your mind. Therefore, whenever you find yourself in a crowded store, you may experience the symptoms of anxiety. Usually this association must happen several times before a phobia develops. Although the attacks of anxiety might stop, you'll continue to experience the phobia, which has become a conditioned fear.

Your mind can play a role in the spread of anxiety and phobias by causing a ripple effect. For instance, if you have an anxiety attack while pushing your child on a swing, you might first develop a fear of swings, and then of parks, and then of wide open spaces, and maybe even of swaying motions. You can see how the phobia can begin with a particular object or situation and then, by association, spread to other objects and situations, even though they may not be directly related to the original one.

A psychological factor called positive reinforcement also can perpetuate anxiety and phobias. The well-known psychologist B. F. Skinner did many studies and experiments to show that behavior can be influenced or reinforced by giving a reward of some sort. For instance, do you offer your child a present or money for getting a good report card? If you do, you're rewarding his or her behavior and reinforcing that this behavior should continue if he or she wants to keep earning a reward. Similarly, if you suffer from anxiety, you probably do just about anything to avoid having an attack of symptoms. If you avoid the object or situation that provokes your anxiety or phobia and successfully ward off an attack, you will feel rewarded by your avoidant behavior. The action of escaping or avoiding the trigger of your anxiety in itself becomes a reward. While you may feel better in the moment for having avoided an anxiety attack, in the long run avoidance actually increases the power of the phobia and you will become more and more afraid of the trigger object or situation. It becomes a self-perpetuating cycle.

Finally, environmental stressors can provoke symptoms of anxiety. Stress can be either direct and external, such as illness, loss of a job, marital problems, and so on, or conflictual and internal, as when you have to make important decisions or feel pulled in different directions emotionally. Environmental stress is less a cause of anxiety disorder and more often an aggravating factor. It triggers, speeds up, and intensifies the symptoms of anxiety, and weakens your resistance to other illnesses as well as your ability to cope with the challenges of everyday life.

RECOGNIZING THE SIGNS

Do you often feel a vague, uneasy sense of apprehension that makes you uncomfortable or fearful? Are you jittery, shaky, restless, and suffering from muscular aches and pains? If so, you may have generalized anxiety disorder, which is exactly what its name suggests. You might not be able to identify a precise cause for the anxious feelings, but they persist and disrupt your daily life. You may worry or fear that something bad will happen to yourself or others, and this might make you extra-aware of your surroundings at all times, even if it means that you become irritable, can't sleep, or have trouble concentrating.

Anxiety disorders involve numerous symptoms that can range from mild to incapacitating. You might experience one, two, or several of them, individually or together. Following is a list of the typical symptoms of anxiety disorder.

1. Shaky legs, loss of equilibrium.

2. Shortness of breath; smothered feeling. If the disruption of your breathing persists or gets worse, you might develop a fear that you will forget how to breathe. To compensate for a shortness of breath, people may hyperventilate, which can cause tingling, numb, or light-headed sensations. When you hyperventilate, you take in too much oxygen and release too little carbon dioxide. A lack of carbon dioxide stops the signal to the brain to breathe. If you breathe into a paper bag when you hyperventilate, you quickly use up the oxygen and begin to inhale carbon dioxide, which signals the brain to continue respiration.

3. Feeling light-headed, faint, or dizzy.

4. Heartbeat disturbances, such as skipped beats or a pounding or racing heart; your heart might take a double beat and then take a longer interval before the next beat. You can slow a racing heart by massaging a point on your carotid artery, which carries blood from the heart to the brain. When massaged, this pulsing point, located in the neck below the earlobe at the level of the jaw, causes a reflex slowing of the heart. You have this point on both sides of your neck, but massage only one at a time to avoid overstimulation.

5. Chest pain and pressure; it is usually a dull, deep ache or tightness in the left heart area under the nipple, although it can occur on the right side above and closer to the center of your chest.

6. Choking, or feeling as if your throat will close or your airway is blocked. This symptom can cause a fear of eating, which increases the anxiety and may cause real choking to occur.

7. Numbness or tingling. Tingling usually occurs in the arms, feet, hands, face, and mouth, while numbness is usually in the arms and face.

8. Hot flashes that can cause flushed, blotched skin; sometimes accompanied by chills.

9. Nausea, diarrhea, headaches.

10. Obsessions and compulsions. Obsessions are recurring unwanted thoughts that intrude into your mind and are difficult to dispel. They are sometimes of an aggressive or sexual nature, or indicate poor impulse control (such as needing or wanting to scream in an inappropriate place, as in a theater). The obsessive thoughts are incongruent with your normal behavior and they might make you feel you're "going crazy." Obsessions often are accompanied by compulsions, which are repetitions of actions in a rituallike way. For example, a compulsive behavior could be excessive washing of your hands or repeatedly checking to make sure all doors are locked. Often the compulsive behavior is a way to counteract the obsessive thoughts you have.

PROGRESSION OF ANXIETY DISORDER

Some people experience isolated bouts of generalized anxiety, and with psychotherapy and other natural treatments, they are able to keep their anxiety levels in check. When endogenous anxiety persists and the symptoms worsen, you might go through a series of stages. Although these stages are considered to be anxiety disorders in and of themselves, they also can be viewed as aspects of the overall anxiety disorder. Be aware that not everyone will develop each of these disorders or stages, or they may develop them at different points in time.

Panic Disorder

Did you ever suddenly, without warning, seemingly out of nowhere, feel gripped with terror and panic? And *not* while watching a horror movie! If you have, you've experienced what is appropriately called a panic attack. If you experience these sudden, unpredictable attacks of anxiety two to four times in a week, you probably have a panic disorder. Panic attacks often occur in certain specific situations, for instance, while you are driving; but they may not happen every time you drive, or occur *only* when you drive.

Panic attacks usually last for several minutes up to one hour, but rarely longer than that. If you suffer from panic disorder, you might go for some time without having anxious feelings and then experience an attack without warning or obvious cause. Generally, panic disorder is characterized by the following conditions.

1. At least three attacks in a three-week period, excluding real life-threatening events or situations involving extreme physical exertion.

2. Specific periods of apprehension and fear with at least four of the following symptoms: palpitations, chest pain, choking feeling, dizziness, feelings of unreality, tingling hands/feet, hot/cold flashes, sweating, faintness, trembling, fear of dying or going crazy.

3. Not due to another physical or mental disorder.

During a panic attack, you feel a great loss of self-control and believe you will do anything to either prevent the attack or hide it. For example, because you feel that you are not in control of yourself, you might fear that you will harm your children in some way; or, to prevent the symptoms of smothering and choking that accompany your attacks, you might believe that you must always eat only soft foods in small quantities in order to avoid choking. Some people will go to great extremes to avoid the onset of an attack, though usually it will occur anyway. Fearing what they may do during an attack, some people become withdrawn or "escape" to a private place where they can have the attack without anyone seeing it. Unfortunately, this kind of behavior only perpetuates the disorder, creates phobias, and prevents the person from obtaining help for the illness.

Phobias

Phobias are intense, unrealistic fears of specific objects, situations, or activity. Phobias differ from ordinary fear in that the feelings are disproportionate to the danger and usually cannot be alleviated simply by knowing or being reassured that the fear is irrational. Phobias can cause enough anxiety that they impact normal daily life and functioning. They become linked to panic attacks when one occurs in a particular situation or place; you might then associate that situation or place with causing an attack, thereby developing a great fear of it. For example, if you had a panic attack while on an elevator, you might develop a phobia about elevators or enclosed spaces. People with phobias will go to extremes to avoid the object or situation of the phobia and prevent the onset of a panic attack. Discussion of the three main types of phobias—simple phobia, agoraphobia, and social phobia—follows.

Simple Phobia

A simple phobia is a persistent irrational fear of a specific object or situation. The fear is so great that it causes you to avoid that object or situation. For example, you might be afraid of heights, dogs, needles, or closed-in spaces. Usually people suffering from simple phobias do not have other psychological problems, and the phobia may or may not disrupt their daily life. For instance, if you fear elevators and you live and work in a city with high-rise buildings, this phobia could be a major hassle. If you are not often faced with having to ride an elevator, however, this phobia would not pose much of a problem at all.

Simple phobias can occur at all ages and are common in children ages four to nine years, especially regarding animals, such as snakes, spiders, and insects. Sometimes

simple phobias can cause anxiety that becomes so excessive it reaches the level of a panic attack.

Agoraphobia

Many people mistakenly believe that agoraphobia refers to a fear of leaving one's home. In fact, it is a fear and
avoidance of being alone in a public, open, crowded place
from which escape would be difficult or help not available. As one can imagine, agoraphobia leads to a very
restricted lifestyle. If you suffer from this illness, you
probably avoid busy streets or shops, tunnels, crowds,
bridges, elevators, or public transportation. Given your
fear of being alone, you might need someone to accompany you whenever you go anywhere. Not surprisingly,
this severely restricted lifestyle can lead to depression and
very negative thoughts about the future.

It is easy to see how a serious anxiety disorder can lead
to agoraphobia. As anxiety builds, panic attacks begin or
continue, and you become more and more phobic of objects, situations, or places that cause you to experience
anxiety. With increasing anxiety and fears, it can reach the
point where you not only become agoraphobic but, in
extreme cases, stay confined to one room.

Social Phobia

If you suffer from social phobia, you have an intense
fear of social interactions, especially with strangers or in
situations where you fear you might be viewed negatively
(for example, on a date or job interview). You tend to feel
that social situations have the potential to cause you em-

barrassment or humiliation. You begin to avoid social situations, believing that it is better to be alone and in control than to be with others and feel anxious or panicky. Social phobia may exist along with agoraphobia or generalized anxiety disorder.

OBSESSIVE-COMPULSIVE DISORDER

Obsessions are anxiety-producing thoughts that won't go away, that the person thinks involuntarily and often finds meaningless or repulsive. Compulsions are irresistible urges to perform specific behaviors in a ritualistic, repetitive way. Performing the compulsive ritual can prevent anxiety and counteract the obsessive thoughts, while not performing it can cause anxious feelings. Obsessions and compulsions are two separate problems that often occur together in what is known as obsessive-compulsive disorder. They are classified as such if they are disturbing and senseless, cause significant distress, and interfere with normal daily functioning.

An example of an obsession associated with compulsive behavior is the idea of infecting (or being infected) with germs by shaking someone's hand. This obsession can be linked with compulsive hand washing in order to prevent "contamination." Obsessive-compulsive disorder is relatively rare, and it affects men and women equally. The particular details of an individual's case may be associated with his or her unconscious wishes, fears, or impulses. For example, hypothetically, the compulsion to check the oven constantly to make sure it is turned off could reflect an unconscious wish to be destructive in some way, for instance, toward a spouse who has been unfaithful.

POSTTRAUMATIC STRESS DISORDER (PTSD)

If you have ever experienced a severely stressful situation or event, such as an airplane crash, a natural catastrophe, a bombing, a physical assault, or active combat in a war, you might suffer from an anxiety disorder known as posttraumatic stress disorder. This illness causes you to reexperience the traumatic event as intrusive and unwanted thoughts and feelings associated with it enter your mind involuntarily. These thoughts can intrude into your waking hours or into your dreams, and the episodes are so disturbing that you might begin to withdraw from the external world. Posttraumatic stress disorder can cause depression, anxiety, irritability, and feelings of guilt, anger, and shame.

Posttraumatic stress disorder can affect anyone who is exposed to sufficient stress at any age, and there can be a time lapse before the disorder sets in. In acute cases, the priority is to calm the patient and prevent further stress. Once this is achieved, the patient can then begin to acknowledge the experience. In chronic cases, the support of a friend or relative can help to soothe the patient, though it is important for people not to feel helpless in relation to the patient, but just "be there" for him or her. Psychotherapy can help the patient understand the meaning of the trauma and to distinguish realistic and irrational interpretations of the event.

NATURAL TREATMENTS FOR
ANXIETY DISORDERS

Holistic medicine considers three levels of a person's being—physical, emotional, and mental—that are affected by illness. Similarly, there are three levels at which anxiety disorders can be treated: physical or biological, environmental, and psychological. In the case of severe anxiety, drugs are effective and necessary to treat the physiological causes of the condition. Natural medicine treatments, such as herbal medicine and hydrotherapy, also can be used to treat generalized anxiety at the physiological level. But unlike conventional medicine, natural medicine also can treat the environmental and psychological aspects of the condition. By learning to manage the environmental stressors and psychological facets, you can alleviate anxiety when you experience it and prevent it from recurring in the future.

Conventional treatment of anxiety disorders includes psychotherapy as well as the use of tranquilizers, sleeping pills, and antidepressants. While these medications can cause adverse side effects, including addiction, they often are necessary in cases of severe anxiety disorders to treat the biological causes of the illness. In addition to psychotherapy, other natural remedies and treatments can be used to alleviate and prevent anxiety. These treatments can be used alone, but are most effective when combined with psychotherapy.

If you think you are suffering from an anxiety disorder, you should consult a psychologist or psychiatrist for an accurate diagnosis. In the case of severe anxiety, panic attacks, extreme phobias, and obsessive-compulsive disorder, medication is often necessary and helpful in alleviating the symptoms so that you can pursue psychotherapy, stress management, and other natural medicine treatments. If you are not clinically diagnosed with anxiety disorder but experience anxious feelings or phobias, natural medicine techniques and remedies can help allay your symptoms while you learn to manage the stressors that bring on the anxiety. Consider the following natural medicine treatments and let them work to straighten out your "twisted rope."

Acupuncture

In Chinese medicine, there is no separation of mind and body. Each of the meridians is associated with a particular organ or *zang/fu*, an element, an emotion, a season, a color, and so on. An imbalance of *chi* in a particular meridian or *zang/fu* can cause physical, mental, and emotional symptoms. When emotions are held over long periods of time, or when they result from a particularly stressful or traumatic event, they can become causes of illness. Emotions also can result from an imbalanced flow of *chi*. Emotions, therefore, can be considered either the cause or the symptom of a disorder. For example, prolonged anger may damage the energetic sphere of the liver, the organ with which it is associated; or an imbalance in the energetic sphere of the liver may result in constant anger or, conversely, the inability to feel anger. This is because each emotion affects the flow of *chi* in a different way. For example, in anger the *chi* rises to the neck and shoulders, while in fear the *chi* descends to the feet. We have all experienced this in our lives: the sinking feeling when we are afraid, the tightening of our neck and shoulders when we are angry.

Since emotions affect the flow of *chi* and you are habitually stressed in a certain way, your *chi* becomes accustomed to that manner of flowing. As a result, tension develops in the muscles associated with the areas of the body involved, and this tension in turn affects the organs in that area of the body. For instance, someone who is constantly angry may suffer ailments associated with having too much *chi* in the upper portion of the body, such as hypertension or migraines.

Acupuncture can be a very effective therapy for the treatment of anxiety disorders because it redirects your *chi* into a more balanced flow. Acupuncture also provides support to the underlying energetic spheres affected by your anxiety, helping to resolve the cause or effects of your stress. From a Western perspective, acupuncture releases tension in the muscles, and this allows increased flow of blood, lymph, and nerve impulses to affected areas. This helps decrease the stress that you experience. Of course, acupuncture also is effective in relieving the physical symptoms associated with stress-related and anxiety disorders, such as insomnia, headaches, neck and shoulder tension, nausea, diarrhea, heart palpitations, and the like. The specific course of treatment depends on the pattern and severity of your symptoms. Acupuncture treatment for anxiety, for example, may last approximately ten to twelve weeks, with one session each week.

Acupressure

Acupressure can relieve anxiety and nervousness as it increases blood circulation throughout the body and has an overall relaxing effect on muscles and the mind. When you release physical tension, you calm your mind; and when your mind is calm, you can gain a new perspective on the problems underlying your anxious feelings or phobias.

Here are some acupressure points that will help release tension and anxiety.

(CV 17) Chest Center

This point is located on the middle of the breastbone, at the level of the fourth intercostal space (below the fourth rib). It is approximately four finger-widths above the base of the bone. Close your eyes, breathe slowly and deeply, and use your first three fingers to apply steady gentle pressure to this point. Imagine that you are releasing tension with each breath, that the anxious feelings are leaving your mind.

Third Eye Point (Yintang)

As the name suggests, this point is located right between your eyebrows, in the indentation between your forehead and the bridge of your nose. Press this point while breathing deeply to relieve feelings of nervousness.

B 10: Heavenly Pillar

These points are excellent for relieving tension and in-somnia that can result from anxiety. They are located on the muscle cords of the neck, approximately one inch be-low the base of the skull and a half inch from the spine.

GB 21: Shoulder Well

To relieve irritability, frustration, tension, and nervous-ness, press this point located on the top of the shoulder muscle, halfway between the tip of the shoulder and the spine. (Do not use during pregnancy.)

P 6: Inner Gate

These points are located in the center of the inner arm, approximately three finger-widths up from the wrist crease. Gentle pressure on these points can alleviate anxi-ety, heart palpitations, and nausea.

H 7: Spirit Gate

To relieve fear, nervousness, and emotional instability, press the points located on the crease of your wrists on the little finger side of your inner arm.

You do not have to use all of the acupressure points described. Find the ones that work best for you, or try alternating the points you use with each session. Practice acupressure for twenty minutes two times each day for a week. If you do not feel any improvement and your anxiety still remains, consult a trained acupressure specialist, acupuncturist, naturopath, or psychotherapist to help you develop an effective course of treatment.

Breathing Techniques

When you are anxious, your breathing may be quick and shallow. This does not allow enough oxygen to reach your organs, and it can cause hyperventilation. Whenever you feel your anxiety begin to build, practice the deep-breathing exercises described in Chapter 4. In addition, here is another exercise that you can use as a warm-up to your acupressure session or exercise routine.

Stand with your feet slightly apart and let your arms hang at your sides. As you inhale, raise your arms slowly out to the sides, palms up, and over your head. Exhaling, clasp your fingers and turn your palms toward the ceiling or sky. Now inhale again, stretching up and tilting your head slightly back. As you exhale, drop your head down and let your arms slowly return to your sides. Repeat this exercise several times.

Your goal should be to train yourself, through consistent practice of the breathing techniques, to breathe in a deep and rhythmic manner. Try to make breathing exercises and relaxation techniques a regular part of your daily routine. Breathing techniques will not cure anxiety, but they can help you to relax so that you can then utilize other treatments effectively.

Exercise

Any kind of exercise can help to relieve stress, tension, and anxiety. By expelling your excess negative emotions and adrenaline through physical activity, you can enter a more relaxed, calm state of being from which to deal with the issues and conflicts that are causing your anxiety. As discussed in earlier chapters, you should exercise at your training heart rate for twenty minutes at least three times a week, if this is approved by your doctor. The kind of exercise you choose will depend on your likes and dislikes, the climate you live in, and your location. For instance, you shouldn't make swimming your primary activity if it is not easy for you to get to a pool. The more difficult it is to get to and do your exercise, the more likely that you will slack off and eventually give up on it. Choose an activity that you enjoy and that you can easily fit into your schedule on a regular basis. Let your doctor know the exercise activities you are doing to make sure that they are suitable for you.

Two types of exercise are specifically geared toward relaxation. One is something you've probably heard about —yoga—while the other may not be familiar to you—tai chi chuan.

Yoga

Yoga is thousands of years old, and yet only recently has the West recognized its therapeutic uses in treating illness. The premise underlying yoga is that an integrated mind, body, and spirit make for a healthy person. Yoga involves not only body postures but controlled deep breathing and a focused positive mind-set. Consider practicing yoga on a regular basis. It is a superb form of exercise for anyone who cannot tolerate stress to the heart, and it will tone and strengthen muscles without depleting your energy or interrupting your blood flow.

Following are some yoga postures. While there are many yoga videotapes and books available, consider taking a yoga class, particularly if you are skeptical at first. An instructor can show you the proper way to move your body, and if you have difficulty with a particular pose, the instructor can offer suggestions for alternative movements. And of course, taking a class is always a fun way to socialize, meet new people with a common interest, and motivate you to keep on going!

Practice the yoga postures before eating and in a well-ventilated room. Make sure that your clothing is loose and comfortable, and you can lay a blanket or towel on the floor if you wish. Generally speaking, you should balance backward-bending postures with forward-bending ones.

Bow   Lie flat on your stomach and grasp your ankles. As you inhale, lift your legs, chest, and head so that your back arches into a bow. Hold the breath for a moment, and then return to a prone position as you exhale. Repeat three or four times. (Contraindications: peptic ulcer, hernia, thyroid or endocrine gland disorders. This is a strenuous exercise and should be tried only when your body is limber and flexible enough.)

Cobra   Lie on your stomach with your toes pointed. Placing your hands on the floor directly below your shoulders, inhale and lift your head, chest, and upper abdomen from the floor. (Be sure that your navel remains on the floor.) Hold your breath and the position, then exhale while lowering back to the floor. Repeat up to six times. (Contraindications: peptic ulcer, hernia, hyperthyroidism.)

Corpse   Lie on your back, your legs slightly apart, arms beside your body with palms facing up. Breathe slowly and deeply, and concentrate on letting go of your tension. You can do tense-relax exercises in the corpse pose, moving around your body, tensing and then relaxing various areas. Once you've covered your whole body, just relax and feel the tension flow out of you and seep into the floor.

Fish   Lie on your back, propping yourself up on your arms and elbows. Drop your head back and, raising your chest and arching your back, slowly slide your elbows down so that the top of your head rests on the floor. Your weight should be resting on your head and your buttocks. Let go of all your muscle tension, breathing deeply and rhythmically, and hold the pose for thirty seconds. Moving your elbows back into position to support you, lift your head slowly and slide into a prone position.

Grip   Sit on your heels and raise your right arm straight up. Slowly drop your right hand behind your shoulder so that it touches your spine at the shoulder blades. Then bend your left arm behind your back from the bottom, reaching up to join your hands. Hold this pose and gently release, then repeat with the opposite side.

Knee to Chest   Lie on your back and bring your knees to your chest. Grasp your knees and rock gently to relax your spine, then lower your legs. Taking a breath in, bend your right knee to your chest, grasp it with both hands; holding the breath, raise your head to touch your nose to your knee, or as far as is comfortable. Hold this position for ten seconds before exhaling and lowering your head to the floor. Repeat five times and then switch legs. After five repetitions, draw both knees up to your chest as you inhale, touch your nose to them, and hold the pose for a moment before exhaling and relaxing your body.

Locust   Lie on your stomach with your chin on the floor, your clenched fists resting under your groin. As you inhale, raise one leg up and hold. (Don't force your leg up too high, as this will strain your lower back muscles.) Exhale and lower your leg, then repeat with the opposite leg. You may be able to do this only two or three times at first, but with practice you will strengthen your back muscles. When you are more advanced, you can practice the locust raising both legs simultaneously. (Contraindications: back problems or hernia.)

Mountain   Sit cross-legged on the floor and stretch both arms straight up, your palms facing each other and fingertips touching. As you stretch up, breathe deeply five to ten times; with the last exhale, lower your arms.

Plow   Lie on your back and put your arms under your buttocks for support. Raise your legs slowly, dropping them over your head so that your toes touch the floor behind your head. If you can't quite reach this far, just rest your knees on your forehead. Your arms should be resting, palms down, beside your body. Relax your arms and shoulders, keep your legs as straight as possible (unless you're doing the modified version), and breathe deeply and rhythmically.

Posterior Stretch   Sit on the floor with your left leg outstretched and your right heel tucked in close to your body. Inhale and reach up with both arms; holding the breath, bend forward, reaching toward your left ankle so that your head falls toward your knee. If you cannot reach your ankle, just bend to the point on your calf that is comfortable and hold the stretch there. Feel your muscles stretch longer, and as they do, try to drop down farther. Hold the pose for one minute, concentrating on letting the tension slip away. Inhale, raising your arms overhead, and exhale as you lower your arms back to your sides. Repeat with the opposite leg outstretched, and then with both legs outstretched. (Contraindication: slipped disks.)

Shoulder Roll   Sit or stand in a comfortable position and roll your shoulders forward in a circular motion. Do five rolls and then reverse to a backward roll. You also can practice this exercise with one shoulder at a time.

Shoulder Stand   Lie on your back and put your arms under your buttocks. Inhale and raise your legs straight up, lifting your hips and trunk to a vertical position. Your elbows should be resting on the floor so that your hands can support your back, and your chin is tucked into your chest. Hold the pose for as long as it is comfortable, breathing slowly and rhythmically. (Contraindications: high blood pressure, enlarged liver or spleen.)

Twist Sit on the floor with your legs outstretched. Bend your left leg so that it is under your right thigh, and cross your right foot over your left leg so that your right foot rests on the outside of your left knee. With your left hand grasp the toes of your right foot from outside the right knee. As you inhale, bring your free right arm across your lower back, palm turned outward; your trunk and head will twist to the right. Hold the pose for as long as it is comfortable. Repeat with the other side. You may not be able to twist that far at first, but with practice your body will become more flexible. (Contraindications: back operations.)

Uddiyana Stand with your feet apart and your knees bent slightly. Lean forward, arching your back, placing your hands on your thighs. Exhale completely, sucking your abdomen in toward your spine. Hold for several seconds, then relax and repeat within one exhalation. Your goal is to increase the number of movements you can do within one exhalation.

Yoga Mudra Sit cross-legged, exhale. Place your arms behind your back and use one hand to grasp the opposite wrist. Lean forward so that your forehead touches the floor. Hold this pose, then as you inhale slowly sit up. Practice this exercise for ten minutes.

Sun Salutation Unlike the previous exercises that are based on isolated movements, the sun salutation consists of a flow of movements. This exercise works every part of the body. Yogis believe that it is important to prostrate oneself to the sun, the universal life force that radiates both within and outside of the body.

1. Stand with your feet together, your hands held prayerlike in front of your chest. Be aware of your entire body.

2. Inhale deeply, raise your arms straight up, hands apart, and lean back slightly.

3. As you exhale bend forward; keeping your legs straight, try to touch the ground.

4. From this position, bring your right leg back as far as possible, bending the left leg at the knee. Support your weight on your hands, left foot, right knee, and toes of the right foot (like a runner's stretch). Holding this position, tilt your head back and look up to the ceiling.

5. Inhale and hold the breath. Now place your left foot next to your right foot and raise your trunk up to form a triangular arch with your body. Your head should drop between your arms, and try to keep your feet flat on the floor.

6. Exhale. Holding your breath, lower your body, keeping your abdomen and hips off the floor.

7. As you inhale, raise your body to the cobra position.

8. Exhale and raise your trunk again to form the triangular arch (position 5).

9. As you inhale, bring your left foot forward and lower the right leg (position 4).

10. Exhale, bring your right foot in beside your left so that you are in a squatting position; keeping your hands on the ground, straighten your legs and raise your buttocks up (position 3).

11. Inhale as you straighten up, raising your arms overhead, hands apart, leaning back (position 2).

12. Exhale, straighten your posture, and bring your hands to rest in a prayerlike position at your chest (the position from which you began).

Tai Chi Chuan

Tai chi chuan was developed by Chinese Taoist monks hundreds of years ago, and according to the Chinese, practicing this artful exercise for twenty minutes each day can rejuvenate your body and prolong your life. Tai chi is an exercise of precise, controlled movements. There are more than one hundred of them using every part of the body, from the eyes down to the toes. The movements are done in a slow, flowing manner, and because they require little physical strength, it is a safe practice for anyone from children to elders.

Tai chi has both psychological and physiological benefits. Unlike ordinary exercise, tai chi does not raise your heart rate, which is important for those who cannot tolerate stress on their hearts. It also has a calming effect on your mind and nervous system. In fact, complete relaxation is an essential principle of tai chi. You must relax all of your muscles and follow through the movements with a calm mind and smooth motions. The movements themselves promote relaxation; your weight constantly shifts from one foot to the other and the motions consist of circles and arcs. Unlike ordinary calisthenics, which usually work one part of the body at a time, tai chi requires that the whole body moves as a unit. As each movement flows into the next, the exercise seems almost effortless, and it encourages a sense of peace and emotional stability.

The essence of tai chi chuan is *chi,* or vital energy, which can be cultivated through the exercise. The *chi* is then stored in a spot deep in the belly, located three inches below the navel, and it can be circulated at will throughout the body. According to Oriental medicine and belief, it is the cultivation of *chi* that rejuvenates and prolongs life.

The art of tai chi chuan requires a commitment to regular practice of the exercise in order to experience the benefits. The best way to learn is to take lessons from an experienced practitioner. Tai chi has become very popular in the past two decades, and some martial arts schools now offer classes in this exercise.

Herbal Medicine

Many herbs have a sedative effect when drunk as infusions or decoctions, and in herbal medicine they are called nervines. Infusions are teas made by pouring boiling water over the herb; decoctions are made by boiling the herbs in water in a covered pot. These herbal drinks can be used when anxiety occurs or on a regular basis to encourage consistent overall tranquility. The general recipe for making medicinal teas is:

4 parts herb
1 part aromatic herb
1 part demulcent herb

Use a total of one teaspoon of herbs to one cup of water. If you use more than one herb, they must add up to no more than one teaspoon.

Aromatic herbs are used to spice teas and give them flavor. Some delicious aromatics include allspice, anise, caraway, cardamom, cinnamon, clove, coriander, ginger, lemon peel, orange peel, and vanilla bean. Demulcent herbs have soothing qualities that prevent any internal irritation, such as stomach upset. Demulcents include arrowroot, borage, coltsfoot, comfrey root, licorice root, marshmallow leaves and root, oatmeal, sassafras pith, slippery elm bark, and Solomon's-seal root.

You should drink one to three cups of tea each day in half-cup doses. It is best to make just one or two cups at a time to ensure that your tea is fresh.

The following herbs are effective nervines, or herbal tranquilizers.

Bugleweed: Make an infusion to soothe your nerves using one teaspoon of herb and one cup boiling water; you can also add lime or linden flowers.

Catnip: This also can soothe an upset stomach, but is most effective as a nervine. Make an infusion using one ounce of herbs and one pint of boiling water. Cool before drinking.

Chamomile: This is a gentle nervine and also helps settle an upset stomach. Boil one ounce of blossoms in one pint of water for fifteen minutes; strain and add honey to taste.

Feverfew: To calm your nerves, infuse one ounce of herb in one pint of boiling water. Cool before drinking.

Hops: To make a tea to relieve insomnia and encourage sleep, boil one teaspoon of herb in one cup of water in a covered pot for ten minutes. Strain and flavor with honey and lemon to taste. To make a sleep pillow, stuff a small pouch or pillow with hop flowers sprinkled with a little alcohol to release the essential oils.

Mullein: Drink two cups of mullein tea each day to soothe anxiety. Since it has a pungent odor, you'll want to add an aromatic such as clover or cinnamon.

Passionflower: This is a gentle sedative that soothes nervous tension and alleviates insomnia. Use half to one teaspoon of herb in one cup of boiling water. Drink the infusion every three to four hours.

Peppermint: This is an excellent herb for an upset stomach or frazzled nerves. Use equal parts of peppermint, caraway seed, and wood betony to total one teaspoon. Infuse in one cup of boiling water for fifteen minutes. Strain and sweeten to taste.

Skullcap: This is one of the best nervines. Boil one teaspoon of the herb in one cup of water for ten minutes. Strain and sweeten to taste. You should drink two cups each day in half-cup doses. To treat tension headaches, combine one part each of skullcap, sage, and peppermint; boil one teaspoon of the mixture in one cup of water for ten minutes. Drink one warm cup as often as needed.

Valerian: This makes an effective sedative and painkiller and is helpful in treating insomnia. Use one teaspoon of powdered valerian root in one pint of boiling water for ten minutes in a covered pot. Strain and add honey to taste. Drink one cup per day before bed. Larger or more frequent doses can cause headaches, nervousness, and vertigo.

Verbena: A mild sedative can be made by infusing one teaspoon of the herb in one cup of boiling water for fifteen minutes.

Nervine Tonic

Here is an excellent nervine that will relax your mind and encourage mental harmony.

4 parts rosemary leaves
2 parts sage
1 part goldenseal powdered root
3 parts skullcap powdered herb
2 parts valerian powdered root

Each part equals one-twelfth of a teaspoon. Make an infusion using one teaspoon of the herbal mixture with one cup of boiling water.

Homeopathy

Chronic anxiety disorders can benefit by treatment from a trained homeopath. But for short episodes of transient, self-limited anxiety, you can use the appropriate remedies on yourself. You'll need to consult a *Materia Medica* to match your symptoms with the remedy that has the most similar characteristics. You can purchase your remedies from a homeopathic pharmacist or order them through the mail. Be sure to store your remedies in the container they came in, and keep them away from strong light, heat, and odors. When you use a remedy, be careful not to contaminate it by touching the inside of the container or leaving the container open.

Begin with a 6× potency and take two tablets every two to four hours. The frequency with which you take the remedy depends on the severity, or acuteness, of the illness. Once you begin to notice improvement, increase the intervals between dosages, and when it seems that improvement is well on its way, discontinue the treatment. If you use a remedy longer than necessary, it might tend to cause the symptoms to recur.

Take your remedy with a clean mouth free from drink, food, tobacco, toothpaste, or mouthwash. Allow the tablet or granules to dissolve in your mouth rather than swallowing them with water, and do not ingest anything except water for fifteen minutes after taking the remedy. When you are using homeopathic remedies, it is best not to take any other medications, such as aspirin, cough syrup, sleeping pills, laxatives, or any prescription drugs, and avoid using any topical preparations, such as liniments, antiseptics, or products containing camphor. However, you should not discontinue use of any medication prescribed by your doctor without consulting with him or her before making any change in your course of treatment. These remedies should not be used as a substitute for any medical treatment you may be undertaking. Coffee also can neutralize certain homeopathic remedies.

The following remedies may be useful to you in treating symptoms of anxiety.

Aconite

Symptoms: Sudden, intense ailments from fright; anxiety and restlessness with complaints; intolerance of pain, fears that do not subside; pains followed by numbness and tingling; faintness or dizziness upon waking up; unquenchable thirst; sudden fever with one cheek red, the other pale; children's croup; painful urination with anxiety; eye pain and injuries; throbbing headache as if there is a band around the head.

Worsened by: evening, lying on the affected side, warm room, music, tobacco smoke, dry cold winds.

Better from: open air.

Arsenicum album

Symptoms: Anxious, restless, fearful, irritable; weak and exhausted; desires air but sensitive to cold; anxiety associated with later stages of head cold, with sneezing; asthma worse after midnight, fears suffocation while lying down; sleepiness but insomnia; thirsty for frequent small drinks; effects of spoiled food; vomiting with or without diarrhea after eating and drinking.

Worsened by: cold, lying on right side, after midnight, sight or smell of food, cold drinks and food.

Better from: warmth, head elevated, hot drinks.

Gelsemium

Symptoms: Nervousness, apprehension, anxiety prior to an examination or public performance; fatigue and aching of whole body; limbs, head, eyelids heavy; headache as if there is a band around the head, scalp sore to touch; sore throat; lack of thirst; dizziness, trembling, fatigue, dullness.

Worsened by: anticipatory anxiety, bad news, effort to think, thinking of one's ailments.

Better from: open air, continued motion, increased urination or perspiration, stimulants.

Phosphorus

Symptoms: Anxious, fearful, weak; associated with hoarseness; tight heavy chest; dry rasping cough; burning pains in stomach, abdomen, between shoulder blades; thirst for cold drinks that are vomited; nausea; night sweats.

Worsened by: evening, lying on painful side, physical or mental exertion, change of weather, getting wet in hot weather, warm food or drink, touch.

Better from: open air, sleep, rubbing, cold food or drink.

Pulsatilla

Symptoms: Sensitive, weepy, wants attention and sympathy; changeable symptoms and moods; craves open air, sensitive to heat; dry mouth with lack of thirst; rich food upsets stomach; insomnia from recurring thought; head colds; loose cough, worse at night; delayed menstrual period with scanty flow.

Worsened by: twilight, rich fatty food, warm room, lying on left or painful side.

Better from: motion, open air, cold food and drinks, cold applications.

Hydrotherapy

Hydrotherapy cannot cure anxiety disorders, but it can help alleviate the tension, nervousness, and other symptoms that accompany anxiety attacks. Warm baths with or without herbs can help soothe anxious states of mind, and once you are relaxed, you can focus on the issues or conflicts that are causing your anxiety. When added to your bath, the following herbs can help soothe those frayed nerves and straighten the "twisted rope":

catnip leaves
elder flowers
German chamomile
hop flowers
horse chestnut bark
jasmine flowers
linden flowers

skullcap leaves
valerian root

When you are feeling fatigued from tension and anxiety, the following herbs will give you a stimulating and rejuvenating bath:

balm leaves
basil leaves
bay leaves
common chamomile flowers
fennel seeds and leaves
lavender
lemon peel
lemon verbena
marigold petals
meadowsweet flowers
orange leaves and flowers
pennyroyal leaves
peppermint leaves
pine needles
rosebuds
rosemary leaves
sage
spearmint
white sandalwood
yarrow flowers

Hot moist compresses applied to the spine, hot footbaths, and hot water bottles placed at the feet also can be beneficial in relieving anxiety. Some people find that damp sheet packs help too. You can prepare a damp sheet pack using the following method: Lay two large blankets over the bed, placing a dry sheet on top. Dip a cotton sheet in cold water, wring, and put aside. Take a hot bath and, remaining wet, wrap the wet sheet around your body. Lie on the dry sheet, wrapping it around yourself, then cover your entire body with a blanket. Make sure you are wrapped tightly, especially around the neck. The outer dry sheet and blanket prevent air from cooling the body and heat the wet sheet within, which thus becomes a heating compress.

Nutrition

If you suffer from anxiety or anxiety disorders, be sure to eat a balanced diet rich in whole foods. Avoid sugar, caffeine, and alcohol, which all have stimulating and depressive effects on moods.

You may have heard that the B vitamins are good for your nerves, and this is absolutely true. A deficiency in niacin (vitamin B^3) can result in nervousness, paranoia, irritability, and apprehension. A lack of riboflavin (B^2) can cause moods ranging from hysteria to depression and lethargy. Vitamin B^{12} is essential for maintaining the proper function of the nervous system. Supplement your diet with a high-potency vitamin B complex, taking up to 50 milligrams two or three times daily. As the period of anxiety subsides, reduce the dose to one time daily with 200 milligrams of vitamin C with each meal.

A deficiency in thiamine can cause negative moods too, including irritability, an inability to concentrate, tension, confusion, hyperactivity, or depression. Thiamine is essential for the proper function of the central nervous system, and it serves as an emotional stabilizer: It can lift tired or depressed people and tranquilize those who experience anxiety. Make sure that you are getting enough thiamine by eating foods such as whole-grain cereals, sunflower and sesame seeds, pork, liver, brewer's yeast, and wheat germ. These foods are also sources of the B vitamins.

Deficiencies in certain minerals also have been linked to anxiety. A lack of biotin can cause panic; low levels of magnesium can cause agitation, confusion, irritability, and restlessness; and calcium has been shown to have a calming effect on the nerves. In order to ensure that you are getting enough of all the essential vitamins and minerals, take a multivitamin/mineral supplement every day.

Positive Thinking and Taking Control

Never underestimate the power of your mind. You may feel that you've lost control when you're experiencing anxiety, but rest assured that you can learn to take control of those anxious feelings by changing the way you perceive and respond to them. Let's say, for instance, that you have a phobia about speaking in public before an audience. If you are asked to give a speech at work, you might try to get out of it, but sometimes that's impossible. You probably will sweat about the event, imagining that the worst might happen—what if you faint, or you panic and lose your voice? The more scary thoughts that flood your mind, the more your phobia deepens, and you might, in the end, wind up being paralyzed by your fear, or you might even become so physically ill that you are unable to give the speech.

Just as scary thinking can increase your anxiety, so can positive thinking reduce those anxious feelings. You can learn how to use coping statements to stop the scary thinking, and talk yourself through the anxiety. First you must learn to recognize when your tension begins and use muscle-relaxing techniques (as described in Chapter 4) to help you relax. Then you can employ the coping statements to change your thinking from negative to positive: You will tell yourself that you *can* handle the situation, and you can recall past successes in similar situations. As you learn to use coping statements and change your thinking, it might help to confide in a friend or relative about your anxiety and ask for encouragement and support to help you overcome it.

You can lower your anxiety level by focusing on the situation or event that is causing your anxiety, rather than on the feelings associated with it. Dwelling on the anxious feelings or fear will only make them worse. If you focus on the task at hand, you probably can figure out ways to cope with it. If it is feasible, you also can decrease your anxiety by preparing yourself for the event or situation. For instance, when you are asked to give that speech to your colleagues, instead of focusing your energy on your anxiety, devise a strategy to help you get through the speech. Rehearse what you will say, jot down notes to yourself, anticipate questions people might ask you and how you will answer them—you might even consider asking some friends to serve as an audience so that you can hold a real rehearsal.

One thing you must realize is that you probably will not eradicate anxiety from your life. In the same way that stress is ever present, anxiety is often unavoidable. But

you can learn to manage the anxious feelings and phobias
so that they do not interfere with your life. Accept your
anxiety and learn to live with it. Recognize that some anxiety is good—it increases your stamina, keeps you alert,
and presents you with a challenge.

In order to work through an anxiety-provoking situation, it helps to break it down into four stages. The first
stage is to *prepare for the stressor* when you can anticipate that anxious feelings will occur. For instance, if you
know that entering a crowded store causes you anxiety or
fear, begin preparing to do so ahead of time. Using desensitization techniques, visualize yourself leaving your
home, driving to the store, entering the store, looking for
what you need, asking a salesperson for help, and so on.
In addition to this visualization, you can use various coping statements to help you prepare for the event. Say to
yourself:

> What do I have to do?
> I can figure out ways to handle this.
> I *can* handle this situation.
> Think rationally about this and stop worrying.
> Avoiding this situation will only make my fears worse.
> I must face my fear in order to overcome it.

The second stage is to *confront the situation*. Remember to stay focused on the challenge at hand, not on your
feelings or what you think might happen. Allow yourself
to feel your anxiety, but tell yourself that you will not let it
get the better of you. Say to yourself:

Take one step at a time.

Focus on the challenge, not the fear.

I *can* do this.

Anxiety is okay; it means that I'm facing this
challenge.

In the third stage you may feel your anxiety begin to
rise as you confront the situation. Even if panic sets in, try
to *stay with the challenge.* View the situation rationally
and logically, recognize that you still can function even
though you are panicking. Breathe deeply through your
nose to avoid hyperventilation, and use the following coping statements to work yourself through:

Stay focused on what I am doing.

If I feel anxious I'll just pause and allow the anxiety
to pass.

I expect my fear to rise, and I accept that.

I won't get rid of the fear, but I will manage it.

I cannot turn back or run away.

My anxiety will not hurt me; I'll face the fear despite
the anxiety.

Once you have gotten through the challenge at hand,
you will enter the fourth stage. At this point, *evaluate how
you handled the situation.* Did you use coping statements
and strategies? Relaxation techniques? Breathing exercises? Take note of what helped and what did not, and
figure out what you could have done differently. Don't
expect to succeed with each challenge—changing the way
you think takes time and practice. Make sure that you
congratulate yourself for even small gains by saying:

I *was* able to do this.

When I control my negative thoughts, I control my fear.

Now that I've succeeded I can do this again.

This gets easier each time.

I'm very pleased with my progress.

I *can* learn to overcome my anxiety and fear.

Psychotherapy

The goal of psychotherapy in treating anxiety disorders is to change the behaviors that promote the anxiety and to explore the underlying issues that are contributing to the condition. Since generalized anxiety disorder is often linked to low self-esteem, a more psychodynamic therapy would be useful. In this treatment, you would focus on your patterns of thought in order to understand the thoughts you have during a period of anxiety. You would begin to question how these thoughts relate to conflicts in your personal relationships, your desires, fears, or trauma you may have experienced in the past. Psychotherapy would help you to understand how your inner conflicts and unresolved issues contribute to your feelings of anxiety.

Psychotherapy is also advisable in the treatment of panic disorder. If you suffer from panic attacks, it is very helpful to identify the causes of your panic and to learn to differentiate between rational and irrational fears, in order to overcome them. In addition to understanding the causes and nature of your panic, psychotherapy can help you to change ineffective coping strategies. For instance, if you usually handle a panic attack by shutting yourself in your bedroom until it subsides, you are hiding from your problem. Similarly, if you know that being in a supermarket or other large store induces panic, you may avoid going into stores at all costs. This kind of avoiding or hiding will not make the problem go away or make it easier for you to handle the attacks. Instead, you must identify and confront the situations or things that cause your panic, and then learn constructive ways to cope with them.

Besides helping you to understand your thoughts, feelings, and ideas associated with your anxiety disorder, psychotherapy can show you how to change the behaviors connected with anxiety that so far have been ineffective in dealing with it. Behavioral techniques such as self-monitoring, desensitization, flooding, direct exposure, and the use of coping statements are useful in treating anxiety and phobias.

Treating Phobias

If you are able to identify and treat an anxiety disorder early on before phobias become too deep, medication may be enough to control your condition. Once the attacks are ameliorated by medication, you can begin to confront the situations that you had feared. If, however, your anxiety and phobias are severe, and even if medication works to alleviate anxiety attacks, you might retain the irrational fears. When this occurs, some form of behavioral psychotherapy is necessary to help you overcome the phobia.

Behavioral treatments are based on the notion that your thinking and responses are learned and conditioned. The techniques, such as the positive thinking methods described earlier, are aimed at reversing, or unlearning, the conditioned behavior. Direct exposure to the trigger of the phobia is key to overcoming it in all of the behavioral techniques. In general, the longer the duration and the more frequent the exposure, the more quickly you overcome the phobia.

Systematic Desensitization   Systematic desensitization is exactly what the term suggests. Using deep-muscle relaxation and visualization, the technique leads you through the act of confronting your phobia. Suppose, for example, that you are afraid of dogs. When you begin systematic desensitization, you would first learn how to relax your muscles on command by using the relaxation techniques described in Chapter 4. Once you have mastered these techniques and can achieve a state of relaxation, the therapist will then ask you to visualize a dog far off in the distance, say one hundred feet, for about fifteen seconds. Then the therapist will tell you to think of something soothing and pleasant. The therapist will ask you again to visualize the dog in the same scene, at the same distance, again followed by a soothing image. You will repeat this many times until you are able to visualize the dog in this scene without feeling anxious.

You would then begin to repeat the same process, but visualizing the dog a little bit closer each time, say at ninety yards away. You would stay with ninety yards until that distance felt comfortable, and then move to eighty yards, and so on. The ultimate image is the dog sitting right next to you or on your lap. Once you achieve this goal, the therapist might take you to visit a dog, first one that is in a cage and later one that is not in a cage but is kept at a distance. You gradually work up to being able to touch the dog and sit with it, alternating the exposure with a relaxation period. Once you reached this point and could stay there without feeling anxious, your phobia would be cured.

Systematic desensitization is a slow, gradual process, and deep-muscle relaxation is important for it to work. The idea is that if you train yourself to be relaxed around the phobia trigger in your imagination—if you desensitize yourself to it—you will be able to apply that process to reality in a gradual way.

If your phobia is recently developed or you do not feel that it is severe, you can try using systematic desensitization yourself. If you do, ask a friend to sit with you during your "sessions" in case your anxiety skyrockets and you need some encouragement and reassurance. Having someone to support you will be particularly important once you move beyond your mental visualization to confronting your fears in reality. In the case of intense or deeply embedded phobias, seek the help of a therapist who is trained in this technique.

Flooding Flooding is a more intense, quicker form of desensitization. It does not incorporate relaxation techniques, and instead of a gradual process of visualization, you would be asked immediately to imagine a dog all over you: jumping up on you, sniffing you all over, biting or mouthing you. You would repeat this scene so often over a period of time that its initial frightening effects would eventually lessen as you got used to the image. Once you learned to deal with—or became desensitized to—the worst possible scenario, you would then be able to face a real dog.

Direct Exposure Systematic desensitization and flooding are techniques that ordinarily involve several sessions. But in some cases it is viable to try to squelch the phobia in a shorter period of time. Direct exposure to the trigger means that you do not have to go through the process of mental visualization first. Instead, you directly confront the real thing. This technique is difficult and may be facilitated by medication that alleviates your anxiety. Here's an example of how direct exposure works.

Let's say that you are phobic about driving a car. First you would begin by taking a ride with someone, watching how the person drives, observing the road and traffic, taking in the street signs and lights. Once you feel comfortable as a passenger, sit in the driver's seat of the car. Close the door, feel the steering wheel, press the pedals, and study the dashboard. Next, with someone you trust in the passenger seat, start up the car and let it idle. Once you feel comfortable sitting at the wheel with the engine on, take a short drive, perhaps to the end of your street or around the block. Each time you go for a drive, try to go a little bit farther, taking different roads, and venturing onto busier streets. If you feel your anxiety begin to rise, focus on the task at hand and do not turn back home. If necessary, pull over to the side of the road and allow the anxiety to wash over you. Eventually it will subside enough that you will be able to move on. Once you are able to drive a considerable distance on all types of roads with a passenger beside you, you can begin to drive by yourself. Again, start with short drives and gradually increase the length of your ride.

When you practice direct exposure, be sure to monitor your breathing and muscle relaxation, and use coping statements (as described under "Positive Thinking and Taking Control") to help you face the challenge. Have courage, persist, and you may be able to conquer your fears.

Self-Monitoring Charts If your anxiety disorder has progressed to the point where you are very phobic—so much so that you often feel it is better to just stay at home where it's "safe"—you can benefit from keeping daily records of your anxiety attacks. By monitoring your feelings and recording them on a chart, you will become more aware of the situations, times, and places that provoke your anxiety. Recognizing your anxiety and its triggers is the first step to being able to treat them; keeping a chart of your emotions also will serve as proof of the progress you make in combatting your anxiety, since many people tend to minimize their successes.

You can draw up a chart yourself, or if you are seeing a therapist, he or she may be able to provide you with one. If you make your own, use an "anxiety scale" that rates the level of your anxiety according to the following numbers:

0 = complete relaxation
1 = slight anxiety
2 = moderate anxiety
3 = definite anxiety
4 = much anxiety
5 = complete discomfort

Now draw a chart that looks something like this:

Time	Anxiety Level	Place, Time, Event, Feelings, Etc.	Treatment/ Techniques Used	Anxiety Level
9 A.M.				
1 P.M.				
7 P.M.				
11 P.M.				

Use this chart to record your anxiety level at different times each day, noting if you are experiencing a panic attack. Briefly list where you are, what you are doing, and how you feel at each of those times. If you are feeling anxious, practice relaxation exercises, breathing techniques, yoga, meditation, or any other treatment that you think will be effective. Make a note of which treatments you use, and then record your level of anxiety afterward.

As you keep a chart like this over time, you may see patterns occurring; for instance, you always seem to suffer bouts of anxiety or even panic attacks late at night when you go to bed. You also will be able to determine which treatments are most helpful in various situations. Self-monitoring may be difficult because it forces you to examine your anxiety rather than deny or avoid it. But avoiding your anxiety will not make it go away; in fact, it will just make it worse. You might argue that confronting your fears only increases your anxiety. While this may be true initially, over time you will overcome those fears. The

more you face up to them, the less threatening they become.

THE ROPE UNTWISTED

It is clear that natural medicine, which advocates that a
mentally and emotionally stable person is a healthy person, can provide immediate and long-term relief from
anxiety disorders. From herbal teas and baths that can
soothe frayed nerves, to homeopathic remedies and psychotherapy to overcome anxious feelings and manage
them effectively, natural medicine treats both your body
and your mind—your whole being. Whether used alone
or in combination with medication, these therapies and
techniques can help you smooth the twisted rope for
good.

CHAPTER SIX

Feeling Those Moody Blues: Depression and Related Mood Disorders

Everyone gets the blues or feels depressed from time to time. But when the feelings of sadness and apathy persist relentlessly, they can be classified as clinical depression. The anguish and pervasive hopelessness of depression is starkly described by author William Styron in his book *Darkness Descending*, which chronicles his own struggle with the illness: "What had begun that summer as an off-and-on malaise and a vague, spooky restlessness had gained gradual momentum until my nights were without sleep and my days were pervaded by a gray drizzle of unrelenting horror. This horror is virtually indescribable since it bears no relation to normal experience."

As Styron suggests, depression is characterized by an overwhelming mood that distorts your senses and perceptions. You feel dark, sad, and hopeless, and events around you seem meaningless. You may experience a predominant mood, such as anger, apathy, or guilt, or you may deny that anything is wrong with you.

The National Institute of Mental Health estimates that 15 million Americans experience a significant bout of depression each year, though only 1.5 million seek treatment at any given time. Depression can strike both men and women, young and old, and it does not discriminate among races or socioeconomic classes. Episodes can last from six months to two years, and they can recur at different times during a person's life. Because of its pervasiveness, depression is known as the "common cold" of psychological illnesses. It is the mental condition for which the most people seek help and the one about which the most is known scientifically. The good news is, depression is a highly treatable illness.

Episodes of depression are often triggered by a traumatic event, such as the breakup of a marriage, death, loss of a job, or physical illness. The severity and the duration of the episode, however, is often unrelated to the reality of the situation. The majority of depressive episodes will abate within six to nine months with or without treatment, but 70 to 90 percent of people who suffer from depression will experience recurrences. The average number of episodes is four in a lifetime.

There are varying degrees of depression, and you may experience a low-grade bout without even realizing it. Depression is a normal reaction to loss or stress, and in these circumstances the feelings of sadness and unhappiness will pass with time. You may feel lousy and blue, but the emotions do not stop you from living your everyday life or rob you of your self-esteem.

You also may be unaware that you are experiencing a depressive episode if your depression is "masked." In this case, you feel only physical symptoms, such as stomach-, head-, and backaches; heart palpitations; or dizziness. You do not feel the overwhelming sadness and hopelessness that is characteristic of depression. Masked depressions usually occur when your emotional state is just too painful to experience directly, and instead you develop physical symptoms. Physicians often misdiagnose masked depression, especially if they are not trained or inclined to handle mental problems. When you visit a doctor or natural medicine practitioner, be sure that he or she takes a detailed family history (a history of depression can be a clue to your real condition) and a thorough physical exam (to rule out any biological causes of your symptoms).

Some people experience an almost chronic depression, with periods when the blue mood lifts. Known as a depressive personality disorder, minor depression, or characterological depression, this kind of depression reflects a maladaptive state of mind or way of thinking. While such people may be able to carry out their daily activities, the depression deeply affects their way of thinking and feeling: It saps their energy and may cause them to withdraw from friends and social activities. The most severe form of depression is referred to as major depression or clinical depression. It persistently impedes social activities, work, appetite, sexual activity, motivation, memory, sleep, and self-esteem. Sufferers' perceptions of reality become clouded by negative thoughts and ideas, and they become even more depressed. The cycle feeds on itself until people feel that there is no way out. Fortunately, with the aid of medication, psychotherapy, and other natural medicine techniques, people can be cured of depression and learn how to prevent it from interfering with their lives again.

RECOGNIZING THE SIGNS

The telltale signs of depression are unusual sadness and pessimism, a lack of interest in activities, and little motivation to participate in them. You might feel irritable or totally apathetic and may cry for no apparent reason. You will know when you are struck with a severe bout of depression, for, as Styron notes, it causes utter hopelessness and extreme emotional pain.

The earliest sign of depression is an inability to enjoy oneself, a condition called anhedonia. Other signals will follow:

- irritability
- a pessimistic, critical attitude
- indecisiveness
- difficulty concentrating
- either insomnia or a desire to sleep too much
- lack of motivation and interest in socializing or participating in usual activities
- great changes in appetite and weight
- lack of interest in sex

Depression operates in a cycle. When it begins, you lose your motivation and interest in things and therefore stop doing them. As the apathy continues, you begin to feel worthless and unproductive, and get down on yourself even more. This increases the feelings of depression, until you begin to feel that there is no way out, that the situation—your life—is hopeless. As the illness feeds upon itself in this cycle, the following symptoms will become evident:

- increased emotional outbursts, such as crying for no apparent reason
- feelings of guilt, self-blame, worthlessness
- exhaustion, total apathy
- neglect of personal hygiene and appearance
- abandoning responsibilities
- silence, inability to communicate
- intense feelings of despair and misery
- thoughts of death or suicide

IT'S NOT ALL IN YOUR HEAD—OR IS IT?

Physiological Causes of Depression

We tend to think of mood as having to do with the mind and emotions. But remember, as discussed in Chapter 3, that the mind and body are inextricably linked. Brain cells, neurotransmitters, glands, hormones—they all work together and communicate with each other to determine how we think and feel.

Even scientists as ancient as Hippocrates believed that imbalances in body chemistry affected moods. While Hippocrates believed that "black bile" was at fault, we know today that changes in the availability of neurochemicals are associated with mood disorders. The major amines, or neurotransmitters, that are implicated in depression and bipolar disorder (once known as manic depression) are norepinephrine, dopamine, and serotonin. Norepinephrine and dopamine are made from the amino acid tyrosine. They tell the brain to get energized, pay attention, fight or flee if necessary. Serotonin, which is produced from tryptophan, tells the brain to relax the body and feel sleepy. When nerves are depleted of neurotransmitters, they cannot relay their messages, and depression results. When there is excessive neurotransmitter activity, the nerves become hyperactive and a manic state ensues.

As discussed in Chapter 3, nerves in the brain and body transmit impulses between cells. The impulse transmission requires a chemical exchange in order for the impulse to cross the synapse, or gap, between two cells. The active nerve cell releases a chemical called a neurotransmitter into the synapse. The neurotransmitter crosses the gap and stimulates the next cell to transmit the impulse to the next synapse. Sometimes the body uses its supply of neurotransmitters too quickly. When the body's store runs low, the person can become sluggish as the brain does not function properly. This lack of neurotransmitters, particularly norepinephrine and serotonin, causes the symptoms of depression.

The discovery of the physiological basis of depression evolved from the development of antidepressant drugs in the 1950s. Two classes of antidepressants, tricyclics and monoamine (MAO) inhibitors, were discovered by chance. The tricyclic imiprimine was originally given to schizophrenics, but it had little effect on their illness. Since it did, however, elevate their mood, it began to be used as an antidepressant. Tricyclic medications interfere with the nerve cell's reuptake of norepinephrine and serotonin after it fires. This means that more of the neurotransmitter remains available at the synapse, allowing for the proper transmission of impulses.

The MAO inhibitor iproniazid was used originally to treat tuberculosis. Since it significantly improved patients' outlooks, it too began to be used as an antidepressant. The monoamine oxidase enzyme degrades monoamines. The MAO inhibitor prevents this from happening, allowing norepinephrine and serotonin to collect at the nerve cell receptor sites, also making the receptors more sensitive.

Both classes of drugs, the tricyclics and MAO inhibitors, are effective because they help restore and maintain sufficient levels of neurotransmitters so that nerve impulses can be passed on. Since the MAO inhibitors produce more side effects than the tricyclics, they are not used as often. Two commonly prescribed antidepressants are Prozac and Zoloft, both of which increase the amount of serotonin available in the synaptic cleft. Antidepressant drugs are very useful in breaking the vicious cycle of depression. Once the symptoms have subsided sufficiently, patients usually can stop taking the medication.

Because every individual has a unique chemical composition, each will require a particular drug and dosage. Sometimes the patient will need to go through a period of trial and error to discover which drug works best. Since antidepressant medications are very potent, if they are prescribed for you it is important to follow your doctor's instructions and to visit your doctor regularly so that he or she can monitor the effects of the drugs. It often takes several weeks before you will notice any effects from the medication, so don't give up on it too soon. If you feel that a particular drug is not working, consult your doctor and together you can decide on the next step to take. When psychotherapy is an integral part of treatment, the efficacy of the antidepressant medications is enhanced.

Studies show that neurochemical imbalances are passed down through generations, and children who inherit an affected gene become predisposed to developing a mood disorder. This does not mean that they will experience depressive or manic episodes; many other psychological and environmental factors contribute to the onset of such illnesses. However, the vulnerability of that person is greater than one who does not have the genetic predisposition. For example, if a family member has either depression (unipolar) or manic-depressive illness (bipolar), the risk of it occurring in a first-degree relative is two to three times higher.

Again, as so often happens in discussions of psychology and the mind, the question of nature versus nurture arises. In the case of depression, certain people are born with the predisposition to developing the illness, and nurture seems to trigger nature. That is, psychological and environmental factors either prevent the expression of the disorder or provoke its onset. The environmental, or nongenetic, factors include socioeconomic status, nutrition, overall stress, physical illness, and geographical mobility. Psychological, or personality, factors include your childhood history and early life experiences, conditioned thoughts, ideas, and behaviors, and whether you are a worrier, perfectionist, pessimist, introvert, and dependent, in which case you are more likely to be vulnerable to depressive episodes if you are genetically predisposed.

Psychological Causes of Depression

Psychoanalyst Sigmund Freud theorized that the potential for depression is formed in early childhood. If children's needs are not met sufficiently, or if they are overly attended to, as adults they could remain, in a sense, "stuck" at this stage of development. If this is the case, the people might have the tendency to be overly dependent on others to help maintain their sense of self-esteem.

Freud also hypothesized about loss, either real or symbolic, of a loved one as being a factor in the development of depression. He believed that everyone harbors some negative feelings toward loved ones, but after a loss, mourners merely turn these negative feelings inward on themselves. Mourners may feel guilty about these negative feelings and also turn the guilt inward on themselves. Normally, mourners eventually can separate from the loss, but this letting go can be difficult for overly dependent people. Thus, according to Freud, when grief goes astray, it can develop into feelings of self-blame, self-abuse, and depression.

In contrast to Freud's psychoanalytic theories, cognitive therapists believe that people's thoughts and beliefs cause their emotional states of mind. Renowned cognitive psychologist Aaron Beck theorizes that people become depressed because their logic is faulty. That is, they distort reality in a way that makes them feel that life is hopeless. They draw illogical conclusions from events and circumstances, and they view themselves, the world, and the future in a negative way.

According to Beck, when children and adolescents chronically experience tragedies, social rejections, criticism, and perhaps a parent's negative attitudes, they learn to relate and order their lives in a negative way. This negative schema is activated in adulthood when they encounter situations that even remotely resemble the conditions under which the schema was learned.

Beck believes that depression can develop because of these negative schemata or errors in logic. There are several ways that a person can misconstrue events and situations:

Arbitrary inference: A person draws a conclusion based on insufficient evidence. For example, a woman might conclude that she is worthless because it rains on her wedding day.

Magnification/Minimization: A person makes gross errors in evaluating his or her actions and performance, either magnifying or minimizing the significance of those actions. For instance, a woman whose child cries a lot may feel that she is a terrible mother; or, despite much praise and achievement on the job, a man still feels ineffectual.

Overgeneralization: A general conclusion is based on a single event. For example, a student who fails one test is convinced that she is stupid and doomed to failure.

Selective abstraction: A conclusion is based on one of many elements. For instance, a man blames himself and feels ineffectual when a business deal falls through, even though many other people were involved in it.

Rather than believing that people are victims of their emotions with little control over them, cognitive therapists believe that people's emotional reactions are based on how they construe themselves and the world. If depressed people, therefore, are victims of their own illogical self-judgments, they also possess the power to change their thought patterns and behavior, and this is the goal of cognitive psychotherapy.

BIPOLAR DISORDER

When experienced as a singular illness, depression is sometimes referred to as unipolar disorder. When it occurs along with periods of mania, in which the person exhibits virtually opposite symptoms, the illness is called bipolar disorder, or manic-depressive illness. A manic episode can occur a few days, weeks, or even just hours after a period of depression draws to an end. Some scientists believe that the manic phase is a defense against the overwhelming negative and debilitating state of depression. As with depression, victims tend to inherit the predisposition to developing bipolar disorder. Whereas there is a lack of neurotransmitters in a state of depression, in mania there is an overabundance of neurotransmitters that overstimulate the neurons. Environmental and psychological factors again play a role in precipitating bipolar disorder.

How do you know when you are experiencing a manic episode, and not just "feeling better"? During the initial stage of mania, your activity will become frenetic and may appear bizarre to others. You might experience bursts of creativity and start numerous projects, though you may not complete them because of an inability to focus your attention. Your mood becomes not merely happy but euphoric, and you suddenly will feel a great sense of confidence in yourself. Your need for sleep will decrease, and during the manic episode, you may go for several days without sleeping at all. Your strong desire for socializing during the episode might result in frequent, inappropriate phone calls or visits, for instance, very late at night. The telltale signs of a manic episode include:

- an elevated, grandiose mood
- frenetic activity and bizarre or inappropriate behavior
- difficulty focusing attention on any one thing
- racing thoughts and rapid speech; though it is difficult to interrupt you, you often interrupt others when they are speaking
- a greatly reduced need for sleep
- increased self-confidence and a belief in your special talents and powers
- loss of patience with other people's limitations and argumentative and dismissive behavior with them
- engaging in reckless behavior, as in having impulsive sexual relations, and activities that have possible negative consequences, such as embarking on a major shopping spree and running up credit card bills you cannot afford to pay

In more severe episodes of mania, you may experience irritability and paranoia rather than euphoria. Sometimes, severe depression can occur concomitantly with the mania or alternate abruptly with it. Delusions and auditory hallucinations can occur, with their content usually matching your predominant mood.

Usually one mood predominates in people suffering from bipolar disorder. For most men the mania phase predominates over depression, whereas women tend to experience longer depressive episodes and less mania. Often long periods in which the person leads a "normal" life separate the episodes, though a person with bipolar disorder probably will experience more episodes than one who is suffering from unipolar disorder. Some people experience difficulty coping with life between manic-depressive episodes and may need continual psychotherapy.

Sufferers may experience ten manic-depressive episodes over the course of a lifetime, on average. Rapid cyclers, however, can have four periods each year, and they are very difficult to treat. Because of the sense of euphoria and grandiosity, mania can be addicting. Many bipolar patients have a hard time adhering to their medication regimens because they prefer the manic phase, or because they believe they no longer need medication once they are stable. However, it is important for bipolar sufferers to continue their medication even during periods of stability in order to maintain the proper balance of neurochemicals, hence stabilizing their mood. Lithium carbonate is the drug used most often to treat bipolar disorder in the manic phase. Once a patient is stabilized, the dosage can be reduced to a maintenance level that will prevent recurrent episodes. Lithium carbonate must be prescribed by a psychiatrist and monitored closely, as it can cause serious side effects. The medication regimen for bipolar disorder, as with depression, is enhanced by psychotherapy and other natural medicine treatments.

SEASONAL AFFECTIVE DISORDER (SAD)

Do you find that you are unusually gloomy and sad during the fall and winter and then spring back to life in the spring and summer? If so, your bad mood may not be "in your head"—you may be suffering from seasonal affective disorder. This illness also involves depressive episodes, but they only occur during periods in which your exposure to light is greatly reduced.

As with depression, there is a biological cause for seasonal affective disorder, and it too involves chemicals in the body. The hormone at issue is melatonin, which is produced by the pineal gland in the brain. We can easily understand the action and effects of melatonin by considering how it operates in animals. Melatonin controls their seasonal reproductive rhythms: Offspring are born in the spring and summer when the hormonal secretions taper off. Light suppresses the secretion of melatonin, while darkness stimulates it. Melatonin therefore is secreted actively at night, and because the nights are longer in winter, few animals give birth during this season, and many actually hibernate.

Likewise in humans, the pineal glands secrete melatonin at night, and light, natural or bright artificial light, suppresses it. SAD sufferers are sensitive to melatonin, and their symptoms increase as the days grow shorter. They will experience lethargy, apathy, an increased appetite, a craving for carbohydrates, and possibly weight gain —almost like animals preparing for hibernation!

If you are confused about whether you have SAD or regular unipolar depression, remember that SAD tends to recur each year during the same seasons. It occurs along with the seasonal cycle of shortened days and falling temperatures. The episode usually begins in October or November and lasts approximately until March. Some people will experience anticipatory anxiety as early as July. Other differences between unipolar depression and SAD are listed in the following chart.

Major Unipolar Depression	SAD
Apathy, lethargy	Decreased activity
Loss of appetite	Increased appetite (often craving for carbohydrates/sweets)
Weight loss	Weight gain
Insomnia/disrupted sleep	Increased sleep time
Deep sense of despair	Sadness, irritability
Hopelessness, suicidal thoughts	Anxiety, inability to concentrate

If you suffer from SAD, the treatment is simple: You need more light. If it is feasible, you can spend the winters in—or move to—a temperate location in which the days are longer. Since most people do not have such great flexibility, there are artificial means of soaking in the "sun" or sunlike light. Synthetic sunlight boxes that use full-spectrum fluorescent bulbs can be purchased for ap-

proximately $300 to $500. Companies that produce the
boxes are:

Apollo Light Systems
352 West 1060 South
Orem, UT 84058
(801) 226-2370

The SunBox Co.
19217 Orbit Drive
Gaithersburg, MD 20879
(301) 762-1SUN

If you do not want to purchase a premade light box,
you can use a fixture that holds six or eight forty-eight-
inch full-spectrum fluorescent bulbs. General Electric
makes a line called Chromaline; DuroTest manufactures
VitaLites; and North American Philips produces Indoor
Sunlight bulbs.

You should seek professional help before pursuing
bright light therapy because SAD often compounds the
problems of major depression. If you are accurately diagnosed as suffering from SAD, however, bright light therapy may be a simple cure for you. Position your light box
or fixture three to six feet from where you are sitting.
(You'll need to experiment to find the distance that is
most comfortable and most effective.) The light should be
in your direct line of sight, but do not stare into it—just
glance at it several times a minute. The light needs to hit
the retina of your eyes in order to penetrate into the brain
and stop the production of melatonin. Most people benefit from between two and four hours of exposure each

day. Begin with four hours, and if you find that you experience headaches or feel jittery, reduce the length of time by half-hour increments until your exposure feels comfortable and effective. If four hours does not seem to be enough to achieve results, increase the time by fifteen-minute intervals. The time of day you choose to sit under your lights is very individualized. Most people seem to benefit from morning exposure, while others feel more relief from evening sessions. Again, you will need to experiment to find what works best for you.

An unusual method of treating SAD is to wear tinted eyeglasses. It has been found that a rose gradient lens inhibits melatonin production, while a blue-green shade increases it.

NATURAL RHYTHMS OF THE BODY DISTURBED

Mood disorders such as depression and bipolar disorder disrupt the body's natural cycles and rhythms. When depression occurs, the brain tries to reset the body's rhythms, but when the depression continues untreated, the brain fails to maintain balance. If the depression persists long enough, the brain eventually will consider it as a normal state and will stop trying to restore the previous natural balance. In this case, depression becomes chronic.

The influence of light on natural body rhythms and mood disorders is profound. The hypothalamus contains small cell clusters that are linked to the pineal gland and the eyes. This is believed to be the area of the brain that integrates daily rhythms according to the most visible environmental stimulus—light. Light travels from the eyes to the small cell clusters through nerve pathways that are excited by acetylcholine. With the help of norepinephrine, it then travels to the pineal gland. Norepinephrine inhibits the production of melatonin, and in the absence of light, melatonin is synthesized from serotonin. The pineal gland, in fact, contains the highest concentration of serotonin in the body. Thus, the major neurotransmitters that are involved in depression—serotonin and norepinephrine—also influence the production of melatonin. Melatonin acts on the hypothalamus to alter the secretion of hormones, thereby regulating some of the body's natural rhythms, one of which is mood. When you are suffering from a mood disorder like depression, it is important that you follow a routine in your daily life—for example, eating, going to sleep, and awakening at the same times each day—in order to help restore your natural body rhythms.

GETTING AN ACCURATE DIAGNOSIS

It is vital, when dealing with mood disorders, to obtain an accurate diagnosis of your illness. Many physical diseases can cause or mimic depression, and milder cases of bipolar disorder often are not correctly diagnosed as such. If you believe you are suffering from depression or bipolar disorder, visit your medical doctor for a thorough examination. Neuroendocrine tests can show if you have any abnormalities in the nervous systems or whether your endocrine glands are working properly. You also should have blood and urine tests and be screened for vitamin deficiencies and buildups of heavy metals.

The goal is to determine if there is a physiological disease that is causing your depressive symptoms. Cancer, viral pneumonia, tuberculosis, AIDS, systemic lupus erythematosis, infectious mononucleosis, and hepatitis are all physical illnesses that can mimic depression. Neurological diseases such as dementia, Huntington's chorea, Parkinson's disease, Alzheimer's disease, and viral encephalitis also have been known to mimic depression. Even certain medications can cause symptoms of depression, so it is important to give your doctor a list of any and all drugs you are taking. Some medications to beware of include cancer chemotherapy, antihypertensive drugs, cardiovascular medication, drugs for arthritis and joint/muscle pain, gastrointestinal drugs, anticonvulsants, medications for Parkinson's disease, oral contraceptives, nonprescription drugs such as diet pills and cold remedies, and, of course, alcohol and recreational drugs.

Once you have ruled out physical illnesses and feel sure that your condition is emotional, you should consult a psychiatrist or psychologist for an accurate diagnosis. Any severe symptoms you may be experiencing may indicate a more serious mental disorder. These signs include hearing voices (auditory hallucinations), visual hallucinations, a belief that others can read your mind, extreme paranoia, a belief that others are conspiring to hurt or kill you, and the belief that you receive personal messages broadcast over the radio or television. If you experience any of these symptoms, you should seek psychological help immediately.

CONVENTIONAL TREATMENT FOR MOOD DISORDERS

Depression and bipolar disorders are characterized by brain dysfunction at the level of the individual nerve cells and neurotransmitters. It is important that your doctor determine which neurotransmitter systems are involved in your case and then prescribe medications that can act upon that particular system. One way that your doctor can do this is by analyzing the breakdown products of used neurotransmitters in your blood, urine, and other body fluids.

As discussed earlier, for more persistent, recurrent, and severe episodes of depression, medication is essential to break the cycle so that healing can occur. The drug treatment is enhanced by psychotherapy, which explores the inner conflicts that contribute to your condition, helps you to understand your moods, and teaches you ways in which you can alter your thinking and behavior to prevent episodes from recurring.

Generally speaking, you will benefit from antidepressant medication if your condition:

1. is persistent and/or severe

2. disrupts your normal everyday activities

3. has an identifiable beginning with symptoms that are different from your normal state

4. is accompanied by symptoms such as agitation, apathy and lethargy, insomnia, extreme gloominess, sadness, and pessimism

5. has been treated successfully with medication in
the past

The two major classes of antidepressants, tricyclics and
MAO (monoamine oxidase) inhibitors, work in different
ways. Tricyclics enhance the brain's mood messengers
without increasing the actual levels of them. MAO inhibitors elevate the levels of chemical messengers in the appropriate regions of the brain. In the case of bipolar disorder, lithium carbonate stabilizes neurotransmitter levels
in order to prevent mood swings.

While doctors who practice general medicine can prescribe antidepressant medication, they may not be as well
versed in them as psychiatrists. If you are undergoing psychotherapy or seeking a psychotherapist to treat your depression, he or she will work with a psychiatrist who can
prescribe medication if your case warrants it. The antidepressant medications are extremely powerful, and
each person requires different dosages and reacts differently to them. Your prescribing physician will start at a
minimal dose and gradually increase it to attain the therapeutic level. It usually takes three to six weeks for your
body to respond to the drugs and for you to notice an
improvement in your symptoms. If your condition does
not improve, or if you experience severe side effects with
a particular medication, your doctor can switch to another
one. Common side effects of antidepressants include dry
mouth, constipation, headache, blurry vision, sedation or
agitation, memory loss, insomnia, excessive appetitite, and
heart palpitations. While this may sound awful, the side
effects are usually mild and subside over time. You should
report all adverse effects to your doctor, who will regu-

larly monitor the level of drugs in your blood in order to determine the efficacy of the medication.

Antidepressants are powerful and effective medications, making depression one of the most treatable mental conditions. However, when the drugs fail and the depression is severe, a doctor and patient may decide to try ECT, or electroconvulsive therapy. Commonly known as shock treatments, ECT has a strong stigma attached to it because of its past misuse. Today, though, ECT is relatively safe. The treatment consists of inducing a seizure by passing a 70 to 130 volt current through the brain. Patients are given a short-acting anesthetic and strong muscle relaxant beforehand to prevent their bodies from contorting from the seizure. Patients awaken a few minutes after the treatment and will not remember it. They may suffer from some confusion or memory loss, but in contrast to the debilitation of their illness, this may not be a bad price to pay. In the case of severe depression, given the risk of suicide, ECT could help to save a life.

Unlike cough syrups or painkillers, antidepressant medications are not band-aid solutions that merely mask the symptoms. They work on a basic level to correct chemical imbalances. After they stabilize your biochemistry and alleviate your depressive symptoms, you can explore the psychological components that have contributed to your condition. Psychotherapy and other natural medicine treatments can change your lifestyle and attitudes in such a way that you can prevent episodes from recurring and live a more healthy, fulfilling life.

NATURAL TREATMENTS FOR DEPRESSION

If you are suffering from a severe bout of depression, you should visit a psychiatrist or psychologist for help. As you begin to feel better, you will be able to use natural treatments to enhance the effects of your medication therapy and to bolster your overall health and well-being in order to prevent recurrences. If your depression is mild, you can take several steps to ward off the blues. Although you feel that you just don't have the energy or motivation, push yourself to try, and enlist the support of a friend to encourage you along the way.

1. Try to look at the bright side of things and remind yourself that there is always hope.

2. When you catch yourself thinking about mistakes you made or getting down on yourself, stop those thoughts. Tell (or even yell at) yourself that you must stop criticizing and blaming yourself.

3. Seek and accept help from family, friends, and doctors.

4. Build a social support network; seek out your friends and socialize.

5. Confide in someone you love and trust; it's important to talk about your feelings in order to work through them.

6. Do the things that you normally enjoy doing, even if your motivation is low.

7. Try volunteering or doing something for another

person on a regular basis; this takes the focus off yourself and will make you feel good about yourself.

8. Avoid making any major decisions until the depression has passed, since your judgment may be unclear.

9. Get adequate rest and exercise; eat whole foods and take a multivitamin supplement.

10. Examine your life and try to figure out if something specific is bothering you; if so, how can you change it?

11. Think about and seek the things you really want in life. Do you feel stuck in a job that you really don't like? Are you living in a busy city when you'd much prefer the country? Don't allow yourself to get stuck in situations just because you feel that this is the way things "should" be. You have the ultimate control over your life—if you don't like something, change it.

12. Try to adjust to and cope with difficult or disappointing situations instead of letting yourself feel defeated by them. Think of your problems as a challenge, and try to work through them instead of running away from them. Dealing with problems and disappointments head-on in a productive way empowers you and makes you a stronger individual.

Acupuncture

Acupuncture can be used in the treatment of depression as it balances the flow of *chi* and blood throughout your body and can help resolve the underlying energetic imbalance contributing to your depression. Since stimulating acupuncture points has been shown to release endorphins and enkephalins, acupuncture treatments can have a calming, mood-elevating effect. In addition, since emotions are held within our musculature, opening and relaxing holding spots can free up the emotions to be dealt with and healed. If you are suffering physical symptoms in conjunction with your depression, such as headache, stomachache, or backache, acupuncture can help to alleviate them. You should consult a professional acupuncturist if you wish to pursue this treatment. If you are seeking treatment from more than one kind of practitioner (medical doctor, psychologist, acupuncturist, and so on), be sure to tell each of them about the other treatments you are receiving.

Acupressure

You can practice acupressure, either alone or with a partner, to alleviate many of the physical symptoms as well as the sluggishness of mild depression. Acupressure is performed by applying steady, firm pressure on specific points along the body. When stimulated, these spots, which are identical to acupuncture points, correspond to and affect other parts of the body.

When you practice acupressure, relax your body and just concentrate on the point you are pressing. You can work on yourself or have a partner work on you. Since depression can occur when you repress certain emotions, such as anger or guilt, using antidepression acupressure points can help to release this blocked energy. Once it is free to rise to the surface, you can examine these feelings and try to gain a greater understanding of them.

Here are the acupressure antidepressant points.

The Posterior Summit (GV 19), One Hundred Meeting Point (GV 20), and Anterior Summit (GV 21) are all located on the top of the head. (See page 280.) Pressing them can relieve depression with accompanying headache and memory lapses. Begin with the middle point, GV 20. Place your left thumb on the top of your left ear and your right thumb on the top of your right ear. Move your fingertips toward the top of your head and feel for a hollow near the top center of your head. GV 19, also situated in a hollow, lies approximately one inch behind GV 20. Similarly, GV 21 lies one inch in front of GV 20. As you apply steady, firm pressure to these points, relax your body and let your tension and depression slip away.

GB 20: Wind Pond

These two points are found in the hollows between the two large neck muscles, just below the base of the skull. Pressing them will help relieve depression, neck tension, headache, and irritability.

B 10: Heavenly Pillar

Located about a half-inch from the base of the skull on the muscles bordering the spine, these points can relieve the fatigue and emotional distress of depression.

B 43: Vital Region

These two points are located between the shoulder blades and spine three inches from the spine at the level of the fourth thoracic vertebrae. They are effective in helping to soothe and balance your emotions. If you don't have someone to press these points for you, you can lie on your back, placing two tennis balls in the appropriate spots beneath your upper back between your shoulder blades. The pressure of lying on the balls will massage the points nicely.

B 23: Kidney Shu, B 52: Will Chamber

Point B 23 is located in the lower back at waist level, approximately one to two inches from the spine. B 52 is at the same level and one to two inches out from B 23. Pressing these points can relieve depression, fatigue, and emotional upset.

Third Eye Point (Yintang)

As its name suggests, this point is located between the eyebrows in the groove where the bridge of your nose meets your forehead. Pressing this point soothes your emotions and relieves depression.

K 27: Elegant Mansion

Located in the groove between the bottom of your collarbone and your first rib where they meet your breastbone, these points relieve depression, anxiety, and breathing difficulty.

Lu 1: Central Treasury

These points are located on the outside of your upper chest, at the level of the first intercostal space (that is, below the first rib) six inches from the midline of the body. Pressing these will relieve depression, blocked emotions, breathing difficulty, and grief.

CV 17: Chest Center

This point is found in the middle of your breastbone, at the level of the fourth intercostal space (that is, below the fourth rib). It helps relieve grief, depression, anxiety, and general emotional instability.

St 36: Three Mile Point

These points are located four finger-widths below your kneecap and one inch outside of your shinbone. They are helpful for overall muscle tone and emotional balance, as well as relieving fatigue and depression.

Practice using these various acupressure points to discover which ones are most effective for you. Once you have done this, consider how you can put the points together in a "routine" or "exercise" that allows you to relax, let your tension and depression go, and feel revitalized. For example, you might want to begin by pressing B 43 (lying on your back and using the tennis balls). Remain lying down and proceed to press GB 20, breathing deeply as you do so. Next move your fingers up to the antidepressant points on top of your head (GV 19, GV 20, and GV

21). If you prefer, you even can rub them briskly to stimulate them rather than just applying pressure. Still lying down, end your exercise by pressing K 27 and CV 17. Once you have pressed all of these points, lie still with your arms crossed over your chest or at your sides. Breathe slowly and deeply, feeling the tension and negative feelings slip away. Your depression is lifting and you now feel energized.

Aromatherapy

As the name of this natural healing method suggests, aromatherapy uses aromatic essences that are extracted from plants. The essential oils are like the plant's hormones: They control its biochemical reactions and relay messages between cells; they also protect the plant from parasites, bacteria, and fungi. They are the most vital substance of the plant.

Most essential oils are clear, and most are soluble in alcohol but insoluble in water. Although it is not certain exactly how aromatherapy works, we do know that our sense of smell is connected to our mind and may operate on a subconscious level. Olfactory nerves are connected to the brain's limbic system, which regulates sensorimotor activities and influences behavior. Smell, therefore, can affect emotional behavior.

Whether they are inhaled or absorbed through the skin, essential oils travel throughout the body to affect various organs. The oils can stimulate or sedate, or they can act as carminatives or digestive aids. Essential oils usually are applied through massage, salves, baths, compresses, and steam inhalation. Massage is perhaps the

most effective since the stimulation of the skin and relaxation of the body help the oils to penetrate. With the
blood and muscles stimulated, the oils can be absorbed
more readily. Warm or hot baths also are effective since
the heat opens the pores and allows the oils to be soaked
in. You might try using essential oils in a footbath—after a
reflexology session!

Essential oils are very potent, and many are too strong
to use directly on the skin. If you use them for massage,
add them to massage oil or cream, and experiment with
the amount to use. Even in a bath, too much of a particular oil could be irritating to your skin. Begin by using just
a few drops. If you like the effect, you can gradually add a
bit more if you wish. Some oils can counteract homeopathic remedies, so be sure to check with a homeopath if
you are using both treatments simultaneously.

The following essential oils can be added to your bath
or mixed with grapeseed oil to use for massage: basil,
bergamot, Borneo camphor, chamomile, geranium, lavender, marjoram, neroli, peppermint, rosemary, and thyme.
You also can use these oils in steam inhalers—add them to
a vaporizer or boil a pot of water and add several drops,
letting the steam fill your room. To keep the steam going,
use a coffee warmer or a special candle-lit aroma pot.

Breathing

When you are feeling tense and your mood is low, your
breathing probably will be very shallow and constricted.
By deepening your breath and keeping the rhythm consistent, you increase the amount of oxygen that is reaching
your lungs, blood, organs, and cells. This oxygen, of

course, is vital for your physiological systems to operate properly. Deep breathing also relaxes your body and mind so that you can examine your negative thoughts and replace them with more positive ones.

You might think that rhythmic breathing is easy to do, but if you actually focus on the way you breathe, you probably will discover that it is not consistent and deep at all. In order to become more aware of your own breathing pattern, try this exercise:

1. Lie on the floor in a "corpse" pose with your legs straight and slightly apart, your arms at your sides and not touching your body, palms up, and eyes closed.

2. Focus your attention on your breathing. Place your hand on your body where it rises and falls. If this spot is on your chest, your breathing is too shallow and you're not fully using your lungs.

3. Now place your hands on your abdomen and again feel how it rises and falls. Does your chest move with your abdomen? If not, focus on allowing them to rise and fall together.

4. Concentrate on breathing deeply through your nose, filling your entire lungs so that your chest and abdomen rise and fall with each breath.

5. As you breathe, scan your body for tension. Zero in on those tight or rigid muscles and let the tension flow away.

By practicing this exercise, you will become more aware of your breathing patterns and habits. Once you feel acquainted and in touch with your breathing, practice the following exercise to learn to deepen your breathing.

1. Lie down on the floor with your knees bent and feet apart. Be sure that your back is flat on the floor. Scan your body for tension and let it flow away.

2. Let one hand rest on your stomach and one on your chest.

3. Inhale slowly and deeply through your nose, taking the breath into your stomach so that your hand feels it rise. Your chest should move slightly along with your abdomen.

4. Practice step 3 until it feels comfortable to be breathing air into your abdomen. Once you achieve this comfort, inhale deeply and then blow the air out gently through your mouth.

5. Deep-breathe for five to ten minutes once or twice each day. Once you become proficient, you can practice the exercise for up to twenty minutes at a time, whenever you feel the need to relax and focus your energy.

Here is a breathing exercise that will help you let go of your depression and feel energized.

1. Sit in a comfortable chair with your back straight and feet flat on the floor.

2. Reach straight up with both hands. Inhale deeply, and as you hold the breath, squeeze your fists so that the muscles in your arms tighten.

3. Exhale slowly and, keeping your arms tense, lower your fists to your chest, almost as if you're pulling down on taut rubber bands.

4. Repeat steps 2 and 3 a few times.

5. On the final repetition, cross your arms over your chest. Your fingers should rest on the upper outside spots of your chest, with your wrists crossed in the middle.

6. Drop your chin to your chest and inhale four short breaths without exhaling. By the fourth breath your lungs should be filled. Hold the breath.

7. Exhale slowly through your mouth. Repeat the short-breath exercise for a few minutes, concentrating on the rhythm of your breath.

Exercise

Exercise is essential for physical and mental health. It improves your circulation and respiration; strengthens your muscles, including the heart; and lowers the levels of fats and triglycerides in your bloodstream. Exercise also provides an outlet for releasing negative emotions, such as anger, frustration, and irritability. By stimulating the production of neurochemicals in the brain, such as norepinephrine, it can help to lift you out of a depressive funk. You've probably heard of a runner's high. The reason runners are "addicted" to running is that it increases the production of norepinephrine, which keeps their mood "up."

As discussed in Chapter 4, there are two types of exercise: aerobic and anaerobic. Aerobic exercise requires the heart rate to be maintained for approximately twenty minutes at your appropriate training rate. Activities such as swimming, running, or brisk walking are all aerobic, whereas weight lifting, muscle toning, and stretching exercises are all anaerobic. While these latter activities increase your muscle strength and flexibility, they do not significantly raise your heart rate so that you experience the benefits of increased circulation and respiration.

Try to choose an exercise or physical activity that you enjoy, and you will be more inclined to do it on a regular basis. You also should take into consideration your schedule and the feasibility of doing a particular activity. For example, if you live in the deep South, running may not be a particularly good activity for you since the climate is so hot. If you have access to an Olympic-size pool, however, swimming laps might be much more enjoyable. Consider too whether you would like your exercise to be quiet time for yourself, or whether you would like it to be a social activity. Many people find that exercising with a partner or group helps motivate them and it makes the activity more fun.

Before you begin an exercise routine, you should have a complete physical examination. If you have not exercised regularly for some time, begin slowly and gradually increase both the intensity and duration of your workout. If you experience any unusual pain or dizziness, stop exercising and consult your physician.

In addition to the basic exercise routine that is outlined in Chapter 4, try incorporating the following exercises. While these exercises will increase your flexibility, tone your muscles, and help increase your circulation, you should combine or alternate them with aerobic activity, or at least try simply walking your dog for twenty or thirty minutes twice each day. Now, if you are depressed, you may feel it is hard enough just to get up in the morning, let alone exercise! But try to push yourself to do it. Once you get into the routine of exercising and you begin to experience its benefits, it will become much easier to do on a regular basis. With any luck, you will experience that exercise "high" and will feel bad only if you *don't* exercise!

Remember to stretch or warm up for five minutes before you start your routine, and cool down with similar stretches for at least five minutes afterward. Wear loose, comfortable clothing and supportive sneakers, and remember to drink plenty of water before, during, and after your workout. Generally, you should do ten repetitions of each exercise, though you can adjust this to suit your own fitness level. All of your movements should be slow and controlled in order to maximize the benefit.

Arms

1. Stand with your feet a shoulder-width apart, stomach tucked in and back straight. Extend your arms out to the sides with your palms facing up and make fists with your hands. Imagine that you are holding weights (or use light weights if you wish) and, bending at the elbow, slowly squeeze your fists in toward your shoulder, then straighten your arm out again. This exercise works your biceps.

2. Extend your arms out to the sides as in step 1 but turn them toward the floor. (Your inner forearms should face the floor.) Squeeze your fists in toward your armpit and then straighten your arms out again. This exercise works the back of the arms, or triceps.

3. Stand with your feet together, knees soft (slightly bent), and bend forward slightly from your waist. Make fists, bend your arms at the elbows, and hold them close to your body. Without moving your upper arms or elbows, extend your forearms straight out behind you. Do ten repetitions of these. On the last repetition, keep your arms extended straight out behind you. Turn your palms to the ceiling, and gently raise and lower your arms for ten repetitions. Both of these exercises work your triceps.

Abdomen

1. Lie on the floor with your stomach tucked in so that the small of your back presses down toward the floor. Bending your knees, raise your legs so that they form a right angle with the floor. Clasp your hands behind your head. Keeping your elbows back, raise your head and shoulders up as far as you can. You do not want to tuck your chin in and pull your head up with your arms. Your elbows should stay back and your stomach muscles should be doing all of the work as you lift up. Try not to go all the way back down to the floor, but just far enough so that your shoulders barely touch it. You want to do slow, controlled movements to maximize the effect of abdominal exercises.

2. Lie in the same basic position, but extend your legs straight up. Lift and lower your head and shoulders, keeping your elbows back and letting your abdominal muscles do the work.

3. Lying in the same basic position, bend your legs slightly. As you raise up, twist slightly to the left side and simultaneously bring your left knee in. You shouldn't touch your elbow to your knee; keep your elbows back and lift your chin toward the knee. Again, your abdominal muscles should do the work and you should not feel a strain in your neck.

Legs

Stand with your feet a shoulder-width apart and place your hands on your hips. Your stomach should be tucked in, your back straight, and your toes should be pointed in the same direction as your knees. Keeping your back straight, lower your bottom down into a deep knee bend; go down only as far as is comfortable for you. Slowly straighten up, though keep your knees soft at all times (slightly bent and never locked). Once you can do this exercise with relative ease, try widening your stance. Remember that your toes should always point in the same direction as your knees.

Outer Thighs

1. Lie on your left side, your left arm bent at the elbow so that your hand supports your head, with your legs stacked on top of each other. Your back should be straight and your pelvis tilted slightly toward the floor. Raise your top leg about six to twelve inches. (It should not be straight up in the air.) Keeping your outer thigh facing the ceiling, slowly bring your knee in toward your shoulder, then extend it back out again. Do ten repetitions on each side.

2. Lie in the same position as in step 1, but bend your

knees to form a right angle. Keeping your top leg level (your knee should not lead or follow), slowly raise it up and release it down. Do ten repetitions with each leg.

Inner Thighs

Lie down with the small of your back pressed down toward the floor and your hands placed under your buttocks to support your back. Raise your legs straight up, keeping your knees soft, not locked. Toes pointed, move (don't *drop*) your legs out toward the sides as far as is comfortable. The movement should be slow and controlled. When you bring them back together, squeeze your inner thighs toward each other as if there is resistance against them. This makes your muscles work harder. Do ten repetitions with your toes pointed and ten with your feet flexed.

Remember when you do exercises like these that your movements should be controlled and slow—you shouldn't just swing your arms or legs. You can use light weights if you wish, or just imagine that you are so that you can feel the resistance as you squeeze your muscles. Although you may be tempted to skip the cool-down stretches to save time, you may be sorry if you do. Your muscles contract and tighten when you exercise, and the cool-down stretches them out again to prevent cramping or pulls. Warming up and cooling down is an insurance against injuries!

Yoga

Yoga is a relaxing form of exercise that can help alleviate depression. It tones the nervous system, stimulates circulation, promotes concentration, and energizes your mind and body. A complete listing of yoga postures is outlined in Chapter 5. The following are especially beneficial in the treatment of depression.

Plow: Lie on your back with your arms under your buttocks. Raise your legs and swing your feet over your head until your toes touch the floor (if possible). Your arms should rest beside your body, palms down. As you hold the pose, scan your body for tension and relax, especially your shoulders and arms. Breathe slowly and rhythmically.

Shoulder Stand: Lie on your back with your arms under your buttocks. As you inhale, raise your legs, lifting your trunk, hips, and legs into a vertical position. Your elbows should rest on the floor, your hands support your back, and your chin is pressed into your chest. Hold the pose for as long as is comfortable, but no longer than fifteen minutes.

Yoga Mudra: Sit cross-legged on the floor with your back straight. As you exhale, lean forward to touch the floor with your forehead (if possible). Bring your arms behind your back and use one hand to grasp the opposite wrist. Hold the pose; then, on an inhalation, return to the sitting position. You should practice this posture for up to fifteen minutes.

Corpse Pose: Lie on your back in a dim, quiet place. Let your arms rest beside your body, palms up, and your feet can be slightly apart. Breathe slowly and deeply, allowing calmness to flow through your body. Let your tension go.

Try the following tense-relax exercise as you lie in the corpse pose:

1. As you inhale through your nose, tighten the muscles in your knees, calves, ankles, feet, and toes. Hold the tension, then relax and exhale.

2. Next inhale, tensing all of these parts as well as your abdomen, pelvis, hips, and thighs. Hold them taut, then relax and exhale.

3. Tense the muscles in your neck, shoulders, arms, elbows, wrists, hands, fingers, chest as well as muscles in your trunk and legs. Hold the tension, then relax and exhale.

4. Finally, starting with your scalp, face, and head, tense all of your body muscles. Hold the tension, then relax and exhale. Feel how all of the tension has melted away from your body.

Herbal Medicine

Many different herbs can help lift a melancholy mood and alleviate the symptoms of depression. Prepared as soothing infusions or teas, the herbs are a wonderful complement to other natural medicine techniques in the treatment of mild depression. If you would like to use herbs, consult your physician, psychiatrist, or natural medicine practitioner, particularly if you are taking homeopathic remedies or prescription medications.

Unless an herb is known to be poisonous in certain quantities or forms, the general preparation is to boil one ounce of herb in twenty ounces of water. Simmer for ten to twenty minutes, strain, and drink four to six ounces four times each day. You can add marjoram, thyme, rosemary, and sage, excellent herbs that can raise your spirits, to many of your recipes. Essential herbal oils such as bergamot, orange, lemon, jasmine, neroli, and rose can be massaged into the skin.

Herbal Preparations

Balm: A member of the mint family, this herb also is known as melissa. Use the leaves and tops when they are fresh and green rather than dried. A balm tea will stimulate your brain, relieving that apathetic, lethargic feeling.

Black Hellebore: Also called the Christmas rose, the dried rhizome and juice of this herb are poisonous in large amounts. It is good in small quantities for relieving both melancholy and mania.

Borage: This herb is rich in potassium. Use the leaves and seeds to alleviate sadness, pensiveness, and melancholy.

Clove: Mix together ¼ ounce crushed clove, two ounces of rose petals, and one ounce of mint. Make a sleep pillow or boil in water and inhale the steam to relieve gloominess and help you sleep.

Fo-ti-tieng: This rejuvenating herb, which has been studied extensively in France, energizes the brain, nerves, and endocrine glands. Use the leaves and seed as a daily tea.

Rosemary: Besides being a great spice for recipes, rosemary is excellent in sleep pillows and herbal baths. It rekindles your energy and will make you feel happy. You can also prepare an effective rosemary tea using a pinch of valerian.

Sage: A member of the mint family, sage has been used medicinally and cosmetically since ancient times. To calm jittery nerves, make a decoction with the dried herb, strain and drink.

St. Johnswort: The flowers of this herb make an infusion that is effective in relieving sadness and melancholy.

Thyme: Also a member of the mint family, thyme is easy to grow in your own herb garden. Add this spice to your favorite dishes, and use it in herbal sachets to lift a melancholy mood.

Tonic Recipes

Steep ½ ounce each of finely chopped poplar bark and gentian root in two pints of water for fifteen minutes. Boil and add ½ ounce each of agrimony and centaury. Simmer for ten minutes, cool, and strain. You can add honey for sweetener if you desire. Take three or four tablespoons before meals.

Boil two cups of water with one teaspoon each of rosemary and sage. Steep for five minutes, strain, and drink daily.

Homeopathy

If you are experiencing a transient episode of depression, homeopathic remedies can be useful in alleviating the blues. These remedies are prescribed based on the similarity of their characteristics to those symptoms that you are experiencing. For instance, if you are anxious, restless, and tired, you might want to try *Arsenicum album;* for melancholia following the breakup of an intimate relationship or loss of a loved one, use ignatia; if you are weepy and feel as if you need extra comforting, pulsatilla can help; sepia can be helpful if you feel depressed and irritable, dragged down by responsibilities and worries. More serious depressions should be treated by a trained homeopath, who can often bring great benefit.

In cases of mild depression, you can use a homeopathic guidebook to administer your own remedies. First you need to "take the case," by observing all symptoms, both physical and mental. You will choose a remedy based on matching those symptoms with the remedy that shares similar characteristics, so it is essential to gain an accurate all-encompassing picture of the patient. As you take the case, remember to observe the following: skin, lip, and tongue color; expression and attitude; the person's body language (the way he or she moves, sits); state of mind and mood; skin temperature and sensitivity; the sound of the voice and rate of speech; pulse; breathing; description of aches and pains; times the patient feels the worst; cravings or repulsions. Take copious notes on all of your observations and save them as health records for future use.

Once you have taken the case, select an appropriate remedy that matches the symptoms. While this book suggests the remedies that are applicable to stress, anxiety, and depression, you should consult the homeopathic *Materia Medica* for a detailed description of each one. Most books about homeopathy contain an abridged *Materia Medica* that lists the most frequently used remedies. If you are in doubt as to which one to use, don't hesitate to contact a trained homeopathic physician.

Homeopathic remedies usually come in tablet, granule, or tincture form, and you can purchase them from homeopathic pharmacists. The standard dosage is two tablets of a 6× potentization every two to four hours. When you begin to treat yourself or others, use a 6× or 12× potentization. If you do not see results, you can evaluate another choice of remedy. Treat with only one remedy at a time, since each pertains to a particular set of symptoms. Allow the remedy to dissolve in the mouth, and do not ingest anything except water fifteen minutes before or after taking the remedy. Once improvement of the condition is established, you can increase the intervals between dosages and discontinue treatment when the symptoms disappear.

Store your homeopathic remedies in the containers they came in, and make sure that you keep them tightly closed. They should not come into contact with anything, including heat, direct light, and pungent odors.

If you are experiencing a moderate to severe depressive episode, you should visit a trained homeopath rather than try to treat yourself. It is also advisable in these cases to use homeopathy as a complement to other treatments, such as psychotherapy and conventional medication.

Nutrition

Everyone knows that good nutrition is essential to maintaining health. But not everyone knows that some foods can cause allergies or aggravate illnesses and that specific vitamins and minerals can be used to treat illnesses.

Depression has been associated with a high intake of caffeine. If you drink four or more cups of caffeine in a given day, try substituting decaffeinated coffee and soft drinks. If you're a junk food or sweets addict, refined sugar may be aggravating your depressed mood. Steer clear of caffeine, sugar, alcohol, and dairy products if you are lactose-sensitive. Avoid processed food that contains artificial coloring and preservatives. Instead fill your diet with fresh vegetables, fruit, and whole-grain cereals, and balanced food groups. You should eat the following number of servings from the basic food groups each day.

Vegetables:	3–5
Fruit:	2–4 (serving = ½ cup or 1 piece of fruit)
Bread, cereals, grains:	6–11 (serving = 1 slice or ¾ cup cereal)
Dairy products:	2–3; 3–4 for teens, pregnant or nursing women (serving = 1 cup milk or yogurt, 1 slice cheese)
Meat, poultry, fish, eggs, legumes:	2–3 (serving = 3 ounces lean meat; 2 eggs; 1¼ cups legumes)

As you compose a healing diet to combat your depression, limit your total daily fat intake to 30 percent of your total calories. Try not to consume more than 300 milligrams of cholesterol a day, and limit servings of meat, fish, and fowl to three ounces each.

If you suspect that you might have a food allergy or sensitivity, eliminate all foods that you eat more than twice a week (for example, wheat, dairy products). Reintroduce one food every three days as it may take up to seventy-two hours for a reaction to occur. Keep a detailed food diary to record which foods cause specific symptoms.

In order to determine whether mineral imbalances are aggravating your symptoms, you should undergo a thyroid function test, urine analysis, and blood tests. Some natural medicine practitioners also perform hair and nail analyses.

Vitamins and Minerals

It is essential that you get adequate amounts of all vitamins and minerals in order to maintain good health and emotional stability. Following are the nutrients that are associated with depression and other mood problems.

B¹ (thiamine): B^1 is necessary for the brain to metabolize carbohydrates, and a deficiency can result in fatigue, irritability, memory lapses, insomnia, loss of appetite, and stomach upset. The people most at risk for a serious deficiency are chronic alcoholics, pregnant and nursing women, people who experience frequent diarrhea, drug addicts, the elderly, people with chronic illness, and people who eat mostly junk food.

B² (riboflavin): B^2 is essential for growth and the functioning of body tissue. A deficiency can cause symptoms of depression. People at risk include women who take oral contraceptives and those in the second trimester of pregnancy.

B³ (niacin): A deficiency of this vitamin can cause depression and even psychosis and dementia if left untreated. Symptoms of a deficiency include agitation, anxiety, and mental lethargy. Those people most at risk are the elderly, drug addicts, alcoholics, and people with liver disease.

B⁶ (pyridoxine): B^6 is essential for healthy blood, skin, and nervous system functioning. It is present in most foods, and a deficiency usually results from malabsorption of the vitamin due to disease, drugs, and an unusually fast metabolism. B^6 deficiency has been strongly linked to depression.

B^{12}:   Found mostly in meat and animal proteins, B^{12} is stored in the liver. If your reserves are used up, symptoms such as dementia, changing moods, irritability, paranoia, mania, and confusion can develop.

Vitamin C: Vitamin C facilitates the absorption of iron and is involved with folic acid and amino acids. A deficiency can result in fatigue, weakness, apathy, weight loss, and depression. You will need more than the standard amount of vitamin C if you are on oral contraceptives or tetracycline, or if you are under stress, pregnant, or elderly.

Folic Acid: Low levels of folic acid have been noted in depressed patients, and a deficiency results in fatigue, apathy, dementia, and depressive symptoms. Drugs such as aspirin, barbiturates, anticonvulsants, and oral contraceptives can inhibit the absorption of folic acid in the body.

Minerals: Iron, sodium, magnesium, calcium, potassium, chromium, copper, cobalt, manganese, zinc, nickel, strontium, selenium, and molybdenum are all metals, or minerals, essential for proper enzyme function. Deficiencies in certain minerals, such as potassium, sodium, iron, calcium, magnesium, zinc, and manganese, can cause symptoms of depression. An abundance of nonessential minerals, such as lead, mercury, arsenic, bismuth, aluminum, and bromides, can mimic depression.

Amino Acids: You've probably heard or read about amino acids. They are the building blocks of proteins, and some of them have properties similar to neurotransmitters, making them useful in treating anxiety and depression. Gamma-aminobutyric acid, or GABA, is a natural antianxiety chemical and is often found in low levels in depressed people. L-tryptophan is a precursor to the synthesis of serotonin, and so it too is vital for combatting depression and maintaining emotional balance. Foods containing tryptophan include bananas, beef, turkey, figs, dates, pineapple, pasta, peanuts, and processed cheese. Similarly, tyrosine is a precursor of norepinephrine and dopamine, two neurochemicals that are involved in mood. Foods containing tyrosine include eggs, green beans, lean meat, peas, seafood, aged natural cheese, seaweed, skim milk, tofu, whole wheat bread, and yogurt. D-phenylalanine is another important amino acid that has been associated with depression.

It is difficult to treat mood disorders with amino acids because it is hard to determine how much of the substance actually reaches the brain, but it certainly can't hurt to consume healthy foods that contain them as a step toward overall mental health.

A nutritionist or natural medicine practitioner can help treat your depression by supplementing your diet with vitamins and minerals, and then, after the symptoms are alleviated, will adjust the dosages in order to maintain a satisfactory level of health and well-being. Since taking large doses of vitamins, minerals, and amino acids yourself could compound your problem, it is best to seek an accurate diagnosis and treatment from a natural medicine practitioner who can perform the appropriate laboratory work, such as hair, nail, blood, and urine analyses.

Physical Medicine

Massage

Whether it involves pressing acupressure points, manipulating the bones or connective tissue, or enjoying a relaxing massage, the power of touch is amazing. For many people, there is nothing as soothing as a massage, and yet it is invigorating too. If you are feeling down and blue, try starting your day with some exercise followed by a massage. You don't have to spend a lot of money for a trained massage therapist (although it is a worthwhile treat!)—you can ask a friend to give you one or you can follow these suggestions for giving one to yourself:

Start with your head and work your way down to your toes. Pour some massage oil onto your palms, and using flat hands, rub it vigorously into your hair and scalp. You can use your fingertips to cover your head with small circular movements. Gently massage your face and ears, and then your neck. Knead your shoulders and vigorously massage your arms with up-and-down motions. Use circular movements on your elbows and knead your hands and fingers. Next move to your chest and stomach using large gentle circular motions. Massage your sides and back, if you can reach it without straining. Again use vigorous up-

and-down motions on your legs, with circular movement at your knees and ankles. Massage your feet—tops and bottoms—and use your fingers to massage your toes. When you are done, take a warm shower and use a mild soap to wash off the excess oil. The oil that has penetrated or remains on the surface of the skin conditions it and helps keep your body warm.

Reflexology

As evidenced in acupuncture, the Chinese have long believed that stimulation of certain points along the body can affect other organs or body parts. Foot reflexology is an offshoot of this theory. The bottom of your foot is covered with points that correspond to various body systems and parts. Massaging these points, either stroking them or applying pressure, releases tension and blockages that prevent the flow of energy and stimulates the circulation of blood. Reflexology also helps crush small "crystals," or deposits of lactic acid, that settle in your feet. Once they are broken up, they can be reabsorbed into the body and the waste can be eliminated by the lymph system.

In a reflexology session, the therapist will massage your feet and then concentrate on specific points depending on your symptoms and complaints. Most of the reflexology points are on the bottom of your feet, though the tops and sides also contain effective spots. Reflexology is easy to practice on yourself or with a partner. You may find that different books contain slightly different "maps" of the feet, so you may need to experiment to find which points work for you. A few points are useful in alleviating depression. A spot in the center of the big toe corresponds to the pituitary gland. Just above and to the side (toward the inside of the foot) of this point is another small point that refers to the pineal gland. In the center of the ball of your foot is a spot that corresponds to the thymus, and on the ball of the foot underneath your big toe is a point that refers to the thyroid and parathyroid glands. Since all of these glands—pituitary, pineal, thymus, thyroid, and para-thyroid—are associated with emotional stability and mental health, massaging them or applying pressure to them can help to relieve your depressive symptoms. Re-member that as with many natural medicine therapies, reflexology should be a relaxing experience for you. If you're the kind of person who does not really like having your feet touched—or you're ticklish—it's probably not a good therapy for you!

Psychotherapy

Although there is a clear physiological component to de-pression, the psychological factors need to be recognized and addressed as well. While antidepressants can work wonders to adjust the neurochemical imbalance in your brain, they cannot eliminate conflicts and issues that are disturbing you to the point of affecting your mood. If something is really bothering you, no medication will make you feel better, at least not for the long term. For mild depression, psychotherapy alone often can get at the root of the problem and help you resolve it. The insight and personal growth you gain from the treatment can help prevent future occurrences. For moderate to severe de-pression, the best course of treatment is a combination of traditional medication and psychotherapy, which can be enhanced further by other natural medicine techniques.

Psychoanalytic Psychotherapy

Since the psychoanalytic theory of depression holds that it stems from guilt, anger, or negative emotions unconsciously turned inward, treatment would help you gain insight into feelings you repress. Psychoanalytic therapy would encourage you to release your hostility, and it would help you to recall and examine incidences of stress and trauma in your life that may underscore the depression. In a psychoanalytic therapy session, you try to talk freely as your therapist listens to and observes you. The therapist will help you to understand your feelings, thoughts, actions, and ideas, and this deepens your intellectual and emotional self-awareness. Once you are freed from your repressed feelings, you can establish more adaptive patterns of thought and behavior.

Cognitive Psychotherapy

The idea behind cognitive therapy is that "you are what you think." In other words, if you think bad thoughts about yourself or you have a very negative outlook, chances are you will behave and act in a negative, or depressed, way. Your thoughts, feelings, and actions feed on each other, confirming your depressed perceptions and creating a vicious cycle.

Cognitive psychotherapy would focus on altering your thought patterns to correct errors in your logic. The therapist would help you change your opinions about yourself and events by pointing out evidence that contradicts your negative perceptions. For example, if you always complain to your therapist (and to yourself and others) that you are a screwup—that you just can't do anything right—your therapist will point out the things you *have* accomplished or succeeded in doing.

You also can monitor your own inner dialogue to learn to recognize destructive thoughts as they occur. When you discuss them in therapy, you would discover how those negative thoughts and beliefs prevent you from experiencing more realistic, positive, and accurate interpretations of events. Once you learn to recognize your false assumptions and the resulting feelings and behavior, you can begin to replace them with more balanced, realistic thoughts.

Behavioral Psychotherapy

Just as cognitive therapy helps to alter your negative patterns of thought, behavioral psychotherapy focuses on changing maladaptive actions and behavior. The therapist would encourage you to participate in normal activities, such as getting up in the morning, going shopping, doing chores, and so on. Likewise, the therapist would discourage you from maladaptive behavior, such as sleeping all day or staying inside most of the time.

Since doing normal activities is difficult because of your depression, the therapist might devise activities that would provide you with positive experiences so that you will want to do them again. If a specific activity seems insurmountable, the therapist would break it down into more managable components. For example, if your therapist asks you to try doing the weekly food shopping and you feel that you cannot, he or she would help you work up to it. First, you would practice getting up every morning, showering, and getting dressed. Once you are able to do this every day, your therapist would ask you to begin going outside for at least five or ten minutes, even if it's just to stand or sit in your yard. Once you feel comfortable going outside, you would start to go for walks or drives. When this becomes a comfortable activity, you would be asked, finally, to go food shopping. If it still seems like a difficult task, ask a friend to go with you for support and encouragement. Once you have accomplished the activity, your therapist would stress the fact that it was not, in fact, insurmountable, as you had feared.

You also can monitor your negative thoughts and behavior and learn to compare them to available information (this is sometimes called "reality checking") to determine if they are justified; most likely they are not. As you engage in this self-monitoring, you can begin to identify recurring patterns and themes, all toward the goal of learning to think and behave more positively and realistically.

Monitoring Your Thoughts

People who are depressed tend to get down on themselves a lot, and often for no good (realistic) reason. During depression, negative thoughts dominate and your perceptions are distorted, often leading to all-or-nothing attitudes that can become very self-defeating.

Although it may be hard, take the time to listen to your thoughts and evaluate whether they are rational and justified or false and distorted. Learn to recognize your own self-criticism when you hear it going through your mind. Most important of all, learn to talk back to yourself. You must replace your distorted negative thoughts and perceptions with more realistic and positive ones. Keeping a diary or log of your thoughts is a good way to become attuned to them, to recognize the errors in your logic and correct them. Your log should list the negative thought, the type of distortion it involves, and your own rational response to this thought. Tyes of distorted thoughts include overgeneralizations ("I always mess up"), all-or-nothing attitudes ("I'm a total failure"), irrational predictions ("No one at the party will like me"), magnification or minimization ("That C will blow my whole grade point average"; "I only got a B—I'm surprised I even passed"), emotional reasoning ("I *feel* so worthless that I really must be"), and labeling yourself negatively ("I really am a jerk"). In the last column of your log, the "rational response" column, don't just placate yourself with your reasoning. Look at the truth and reality of the situation and write a response that you really believe. Recording your negative thoughts in this way can help you view them more objectively. You get them out of your head and on paper where you can look at them, think about them, and come up with responses to refute them. Writing down your thoughts and feelings in this way helps a great deal. An excellent book that explores this technique in depth is *Feeling Good* by Dr. David Burns.

Monitoring Your Behavior

If your depression has gotten you so down that you are withdrawn and feel almost paralyzed about doing the things you normally would do, it might help to keep a chart or log of your activities. This does not mean the activities you do—which may not be very much at all—but the things you would like to do and the things that you plan for each day. Draw up a day-by-day chart, or use a daily planner book, to record the activities you plan for morning, afternoon, and evening. If you are severely depressed and often don't even get dressed, write in even the smallest tasks, such as showering and eating meals. Next to this list, check off the activities you actually do and note whether they were chores (such as going to the store or cleaning your house) or pleasure activities (such as reading a book or going to a movie). Try to work on those activities that you cannot seem to get around to. For example, if going to the store keeps getting pushed off from one day to the next, try to figure out why you are avoiding this task. Then devise a strategy to work up to the chore. If going out in public makes you nervous, practice stepping outside for just a few minutes each day, then lengthening the time as you grow more comfortable with it. Then begin taking walks and going for drives, perhaps going to a public place where there usually are not many people. Eventually you will realize that your fears and negative thoughts were irrational—by working up to the task you are proving them to be so—and you will feel able to go to the store.

Depression is characterized by a great lack of motivation. You don't see the point in doing certain things and you'll probably just mess up anyway, right? Wrong. In fact, if you stop to examine the things you put off doing and then do them, you probably will find that (1) they were not so hard to do, (2) it really was worth trying, and

(3) you succeeded! Keep a chart of the activities you feel you are procrastinating on. Using percentages, rate how difficult you think the task will be and also how satisfying it would be to do the task. Now give the activity a shot. Once you've done it, record how difficult it actually was and the satisfaction you got from doing it. Do you notice any discrepancies? You also can make pro and con lists when you find yourself procrastinating. For example, you would like to tackle the report you need to do for work but keep putting it off. Make a list of the reasons why you don't feel like doing it; examine this list and note which reasons are irrational or due to distorted negative thoughts. Now make a list of the reasons you should do the report. Most likely you will be able to see that your reasons for procrastinating are irrational, but the reasons for doing it are realistic. Face the project head-on, and when you are done, you probably will feel very satisfied. Again, by keeping track of the activities you would like to do and your success at doing them, you will begin to dispel the negative thoughts that stop you from acting and you will find it easier to accomplish more.

Relaxation Techniques

Meditation

Meditating can be beneficial in relieving mild episodes of depression. It has a very calming affect, helps to ease tension, and improves your capacity to concentrate. As you meditate, you also become much more attuned to your inner feelings and sensations, achieving a heightened state of awareness. Rather than dwelling on the negative emotions that are making you feel depressed, you can transcend them through meditation. This kind of personal growth, in which you gain a higher level of consciousness and greater awareness of yourself, can help to bolster your self-confidence, esteem, and peace of mind. Your mind is free to travel beyond the busy chatter of thoughts to a silent, tranquil place. In turn, a positive emotional outlook and sense of well-being can help you maintain good physical and mental health.

Learning to meditate is not an easy process. Some people have great difficulty concentrating and may feel that it's just not working. You should not give up too soon, though. Effective meditation takes a lot of practice. It is good to set aside a special time each day that you will meditate, and it often helps to ask the support of a friend, spouse, relative, or doctor who can motivate you to stick with it.

When you meditate, sit in a comfortable position in a quiet room. Close your eyes and try to empty your mind of all extraneous thoughts. Some people find it helpful to repeat, either aloud or to themselves, a mantra. This is a word or phrase that, when repeated over and over, is soothing to you. For instance, you could repeat the word "one" or "calm." This chanting has a somewhat hypnotic effect and helps you to focus merely on that word, thereby voiding your mind of other thoughts. You also can clear your mind by focusing on your breathing. Inhale deeply and slowly to the count of two, and exhale to the count of four. Focus on maintaining the rhythm of your breathing, and visualize the flow of air into and out of your body.

A state of pure awareness, in which the mind is free from thought, allows you to find moments of clarity when you feel happy and free rather than plagued by depression. If you meditate consistently, these moments will grow longer and eventually will become a normal state of existence. You will realize that this tranquil state exists within you at all times, and you merely become distracted from it by negative thoughts and illness. By practicing meditation, you can transcend the negative feelings, and eventually they will fall away of their own accord.

If you find it difficult to meditate, try making a tape recording of the following exercise. This will help you relax, and once you are able to achieve this state of relaxation at will, it might be easier for you to meditate. When you record this, be sure to speak in a slow, even tone, allowing pauses between each sentence so you have ample time to follow and feel each instruction.

Close your eyes and let your limbs hang loose and free. . . . Let your shoulders drop. . . . Feel the tension release from your head and neck. . . . Take deep breaths in. . . . Feel the air filling your lungs. . . . Exhale slowly. . . . Feel your forehead and face muscles relax. . . . Let the frown lines slip away. . . . Feel your shoulders relax and the tension disappear from your back. . . . Remember to keep breathing, slowly, deeply. . . . Focus on the air moving in and out. . . . Let go of the tension and feel your body grow warm and heavy. . . . Your arms are limp and comfortable. . . . Feel the blood flowing through your body down to your fingers and toes. . . . You may feel a tingling sensation. . . . Your legs are also limp. . . . Feel them grow heavy and warm as the blood flows through them. . . . Continue to breathe deeply. . . . Let the tension flow away and the comfort and warmth take over your body. . . . The room is dim and quiet. . . . Your mind is emptied of all thoughts. . . . You feel at peace. . . . Continue to breathe, inhale and exhale. . . . Continue to feel relaxed and calm. . . . When you are ready, slowly become aware of your presence in the room. . . . When you are ready, slowly open your eyes. . . . Continue to feel relaxed, calm. . . . Take your warmth and comfort with you. . . . You are refreshed and calm.

Choose a special time of day to listen to your tape, one that is likely to be quiet and uninterrupted for you. Put on your answering machine, turn off all radios and televisions and even the ringer on your phone. This will ensure that you are not jolted by any extraneous noise. You probably will find that practicing this relaxation exercise is both soothing and refreshing. It is an easy, cost-free therapy to combine with other treatments in the treatment of depression.

Feeling Your Spirits Rise

Your health—and life—may seem hopeless when you are in the grips of depression, but remember that it is a highly treatable disease and, therefore, often a temporary episode in your life. You must acknowledge your illness before you can begin to help yourself, and if you simply cannot face your depression alone, by all means seek help. A natural medicine practitioner from any of the holistic disciplines can help lift you out of the blues. And once your depression subsides, you can maintain these natural therapies and remedies as a defense against recurrences. Making natural medicine part of your overall plan for good health will ensure that you are living the healthiest, most fulfilling life possible.

GLOSSARY

anhedonia: An inability to experience pleasure.

antidepressant: A medication used to treat depression.

anxiety disorders: Psychological disorders that involve excessive levels of negative emotions such as nervousness, tension, worry, fright, and anxiety.

autonomic nervous system: Nervous system that controls involuntary actions of internal organs, such as heartbeat, and is important in the experience of emotions.

axons: Parts of neurons that transmit messages to synapses.

behavioral psychotherapy: Psychotherapy in which the therapist helps the client replace maladaptive or abnormal actions with adaptive behavior.

bipolar disorder: Condition in which there are alternating episodes of depression and mania, also called manic-depression.

catecholamines: Neurotransmitters that have an activating function, including norepinephrine, epinephrine, and dopamine.

cognitive psychotherapy: Psychotherapy that teaches the client new, more adaptive ways of thinking and perceiving situations and events.

coping mechanisms: Specific ways of coping with conflict and stress and one's reaction to it.

dendrites: Branches extending from the neuron that receive messages from other neurons.

desensitization: Behavioral therapy in which the client uses visualization and relaxation techniques to confront the object of the phobia in gradual stages (from least frightening aspects to most frightening) until the fear is overcome.

dopamine: Neurotransmitter present in areas of the brain that control motor action; tells brain to become alert and energized, ready for fight or flight.

endocrine system: System of glands that produces hormones.

endorphins: Opiates, or substances that reduce pain, that are produced in the body.

flooding: Behavioral therapy in which the client is confronted with high levels of the object of the phobia until the fear is overcome.

hormones: Chemicals produced by endocrine glands that control internal organs.

insomnia: Chronic inability to sleep.

mania: Disturbance of mood in which one experiences euphoria, unrealistic optimism, and heightened sensory pleasures.

monoamine oxidase (MAO) inhibitors: A class of antidepressant medications that inhibit the enzyme called monoamine oxidase, which breaks down norepinephrine in the synapse.

nervine: An agent that calms or sedates.

neuroleptics: Drugs that reduce psychotic symptoms but have side effects resembling symptoms of neurological disease.

neuron: Nerve cell.

neurotransmitter: Chemical in the brain that facilitates passage of messages or impulses from one neuron to the next.

norepinephrine: Neurotransmitter that tells the brain to become alert and energized, ready for fight or flight.

obsessive-compulsive disorder: Disorder that involves persistent anxiety-provoking thoughts and irresitible urges to engage in specific repetitive behavior.

panic disorder: Disorder in which calm periods are broken by very intense attacks of anxiety.

parasympathetic nervous system: Part of the autonomic nervous system that generally calms internal organs.

phobia: A persistent, intense, irrational fear of something specific.

posttraumatic stress disorder: Disorder in which one experiences intense flashbacks of a past trauma.

psychoanalytic psychotherapy: Based on Freud's theory that psychological problems are caused by unconscious conflicts, this therapy helps the client explore his or her unconscious conflicts.

psychosomatic illness: Physical illness that is psychological rather than biological in origin.

seasonal affective disorder (SAD): Episodes of depression experienced along with the seasonal cycle of shortened days and lowered temperatures.

serotonin: Neurotransmitter that tells the brain to relax the body.

sympathetic nervous system: Part of the autonomic nervous system that generally activates internal organs during emotional arousal.

synapse: The gap between neurons.

tricyclic: One group of antidepressants whose molecular structure consists of three rings. These drugs interfere with the reuptake of norepinephrine and serotonin after the neuron has fired.

unipolar depression: Depression that is experienced without the alternation of manic episodes.

Natural Medicine Resources

American Association of Acupuncture and Oriental Medicine
4101 Lake Boone Trail
Suite 201
Raleigh, NC 27607-6528
(919) 965-7546

American Association of Naturopathic Physicians
P.O. Box 2579
Kirkland, WA 98083-2579
(206) 827-6035

American Association of Orthomolecular Medicine
900 North Federal Highway
Suite 330
Boca Raton, FL 33432
(407) 276-6167

American Chiropractic Association
17 Clarendon Boulevard
Arlington, VA 22209
(703) 276-8800

American Foundation for Alternative Health Care, Research and Development
25 Landfield Avenue

Monticello, NY 12701
(914) 794-8181

American Holistic Medical Association
2727 Fairview Avenue East
Suite B
Seattle, WA 98102
(206) 322-6842

American Massage Therapy Association
National Information Office
1130 West North Shore Avenue
Chicago, IL 60626
(312) 761-2682

American Mental Health Foundation
2 East 86th Street
New York, NY 10024
(212) 737-9029

The American Society of Clinical Hypnosis
2400 East Devon Avenue
Des Plaines, IL 60018
(708) 297-3317

**Association for Applied Psychophysiology and Bio-
feedback**
10200 West 44 Avenue
Wheat Ridge, CO 80033
(303) 422-8436

Association for Humanistic Psychology
325 Ninth Street
San Francisco, CA 90035
(415) 346-3246

Biofeedback Certification Institute of America
10200 West 44 Avenue 304
Wheat Ridge, CO 80033
(303) 420-2902

Biofeedback Research Institute, Inc.
6399 Wilshire Boulevard, Suite 1010
Los Angeles, CA 90048
(213) 933-9451

Center for Medical Consumers
237 Thompson Street
New York, NY 10012
(212) 674-7105

Human Nutrition Center
6303 Ivy Lane
Greenbelt, MD 20770
(301) 344-2340

International Academy of Nutrition and Preventive Medicine
P.O. Box 5832
Lincoln, NE 68505
(402) 467-2716

International Institute of Reflexology
P.O. Box 12462
St. Petersburg, FL 33733
(813) 343-4811

Integral Yoga Institute
227 West 13th Street
New York, NY 10011
(212) 929-0586

National Accreditation Commission for Schools and Colleges of Acupuncture and Oriental Medicine
8403 Colesville Road
Suite 370
Silver Spring, MD 20919
(301) 608-9680

National Alliance for the Mentally Ill
200 North Glebe Road
Arlington, VA 22203-3754
(703) 524-7600
(800) 950-6264

National Center for Homeopathy
801 North Fairfax
Suite 306
Alexandria, VA 22314
(703) 548-7790

National Commission for the Certification of Acupuncturists
1424 16 Street NW, Suite 501
Washington, DC 20036
(202) 232-1404

National Depressive and Manic Depressive Association
Merchandise Mart Box 3395
Chicago, IL 60654
(312) 446-9009

Herb Sources

Annandale Apothecary
7023 Little River Turnpike
Annandale, VA 22003

Boerick and Tafel, Inc.
1011 Arch Street
Philadelphia, PA 19107
or
2381 Circadian Way
Santa Rosa, CA 95407

Boiron-Borneman, Inc.
6 Campus Blvd.
Newton Square, PA 19073

Ehrhart and Karl
17 North Wabash Avenue
Chicago, IL 60602

Herbarium
264 Exchange Street
Chicopee, MA

Horton and Converse
621 West Pico Blvd.
Los Angeles, CA 90015

Humphreys Pharmacal Company
63 Meadow Road
Rutherford, NJ 07070

Keihl Pharmacy, Inc.
109 Third Avenue
New York, NY 10003

Luyties Pharmacal Company
4200 Laclede Avenue
St. Louis, MO 63108

Mylans Homeopathic Pharmacy
222 O'Farrell Street
San Francisco, CA 94102

Running Fox Farm (flower essences)
74 Thrashing Hill Road
Worthington, MA 01098
(413) 238-4291

Santa Monica Drug
1513 Fourth Street
Santa Monica, CA 90401

Standard Homeopathic Company
204–210 West 131 Street
Los Angeles, CA 90061

Washington Homeopathic Pharmacy
4914 Delray Avenue
Bethesda, MD 20814

Weleda, Inc.
841 South Main Street
Spring Valley, NY 10977

Acupressure Points

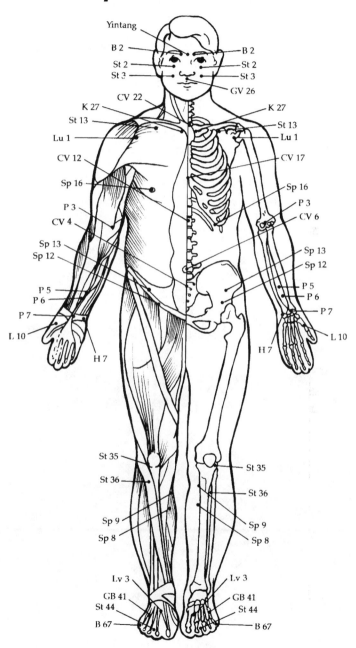

Front View

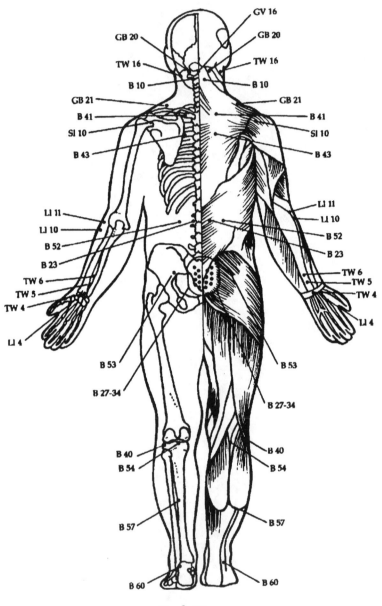

GV 16

GB 20   GB 20

TW 16   TW 16

B 10   B 10

GB 21   GB 21

B 41   B 41

SI 10   SI 10

B 43   B 43

LI 11   LI 11

LI 10   LI 10

B 52   B 52

B 23   B 23

TW 6   TW 6

TW 5   TW 5

TW 4   TW 4

LI 4   LI 4

B 53   B 53

B 27-34   B 27-34

B 40   B 40

B 54   B 54

B 57   B 57

B 60   B 60

Back View

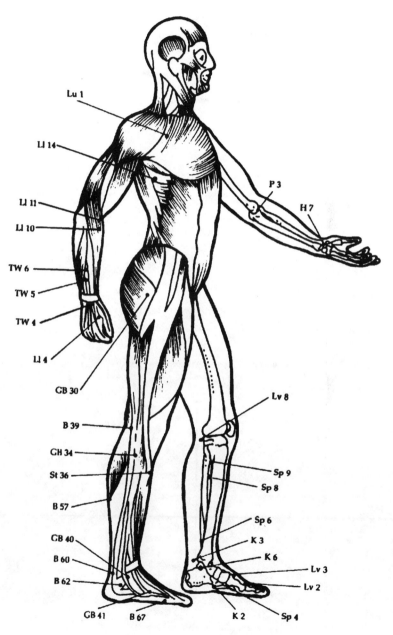

Side View

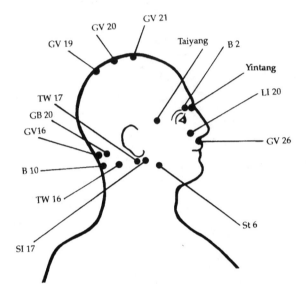

Side View—Head

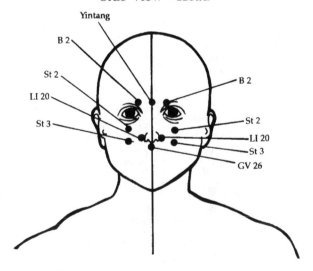

Front View—Head

The Natural Medicine Collective:

BIOGRAPHIES

Dr. William Bergman *(Homeopathy)*

William Bergman holds an M.D. degree from Columbia University and has completed postgraduate physicians' programs sponsored by the National Center for Homeopathy, the International Foundation for Homeopathy, and the United States Homeopathic Association. He is the medical director of Hahnemann Health Associates, one of the most comprehensive homeopathic medical and educational facilities in New York. Dr. Bergman also serves as the president of the World Medical Health Foundation, Inc., an organization researching the cause, treatment, and prevention of disease.

Brian Clement *(Nutrition)*

Brian Clement is the director of the Hippocrates Institute, the first progressive health center in this country. A founding director of the Coalition of Holistic Health, he has served as director at health centers in Denmark and Greece and has consulted at holistic clinics throughout the world. With more than twenty years of international leadership experience in the field of alternative health care, he has appeared on numerous radio and television shows and has conducted hundreds of workshops and seminars on natural medicine.

Dr. Brian Fradet *(Chiropractic, Panel Coordinator)*

Brian Fradet holds a doctorate of chiropractic from the prestigious New York Chiropractic College and has completed postgraduate research in neurology at the New York University Medical Center. He is a long-standing member of the American Chiropractic Association, the Foundation for Chiropractic Education and Research, the Parker Chiropractic Research Foundation, the New York State Chiropractic Association, and the Chiropractic Federated Society of New York. He is the founder of the Fradet Pain Clinic in New York.

Elaine Retholtz, L.Ac. *(Acupuncture)*

Elaine Retholtz is a licensed acupuncturist and a diplomate of the National Commission for the Certification of Acupuncturists. She is a graduate of the Tri-State Institute of Traditional Chinese Acupuncture. She holds a master's degree in nutritional sciences from the University of Wisconsin–Madison. She maintains a private practice in New York specializing in acupuncture. She is the supervising acupuncturist for Crossroads: An Alternative for Women Offenders— A Project of the Center for Community Alternatives (formerly National Center on Institutions and Alternatives/ Northeast).

Dr. James Lawrence Thomas *(Psychology)*

James Lawrence Thomas is a licensed psychologist and neuropsychologist with postdoctoral certificates in cognitive, relationship, group, and brief therapy. He is on the faculty of the New York University Medical Center and has served as the consulting neuropsychologist to Mt. Sinai Medical Center's Department of Neurology. He holds degrees from Yale, the University of California, Berkeley, and City University of New York. Dr. Thomas maintains a private practice in New York.

Dr. Maurice H. Werness, Jr. *(Naturopathy)*

Maurice H. Werness, Jr., received a doctoral degree from the Bastyr College of Naturopathic Medicine. He is the medical director of Healingheart Healthcare, one of the West Coast's most prominent facilities for holistic care. He is also the director of development at the Institute for Naturopathic Medicine. A former tennis professional, Dr. Werness is the founder and director of True Tennis, an organization that teaches tennis and health education to physically and emotionally challenged people.

Diana L. Ajjan is a freelance writer specializing in health issues. She lives in Northampton, Massachusetts.

Index

Printed in the United States
by Baker & Taylor Publisher Services